# Practical Management of
# DIABETES

# Practical Management of DIABETES

**Ajit B Kumthekar** MD
Member
Research Society for the Study of Diabetes in India (RSSDI)
Joint Secretary of Maharashtra Chapter of RSSDI
Maharashtra, India

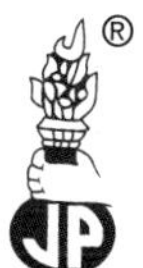


JAYPEE BROTHERS MEDICAL PUBLISHERS (P) LTD

Mumbai • St Louis (USA) • Panama City (Panama) • London (UK) • New Delhi • Ahmedabad
Bengaluru • Chennai • Hyderabad • Kochi • Kolkata • Lucknow • Nagpur

*Published by*
Jitendar P Vij
**Jaypee Brothers Medical Publishers (P) Ltd**
***Corporate Office***
4838/24 Ansari Road, Daryaganj, **New Delhi** - 110002, India
Phone: +91-11-43574357, Fax: +91-11-43574314

***Registered Office***
B-3 EMCA House, 23/23B Ansari Road, Daryaganj, **New Delhi** - 110 002, India
Phones: +91-11-23272143, +91-11-23272703, +91-11-23282021, +91-11-23245672
Rel: +91-11-32558559, Fax: +91-11-23276490, +91-11-23245683
e-mail: jaypee@jaypeebrothers.com, Website: www.jaypeebrothers.com

***Offices in India***
- **Ahmedabad**, Phone: Rel: +91-79-32988717, e-mail: ahmedabad@jaypeebrothers.com
- **Bengaluru**, Phone: Rel: +91-80-32714073, e-mail: bangalore@jaypeebrothers.com
- **Chennai**, Phone: Rel: +91-44-32972089, e-mail: chennai@jaypeebrothers.com
- **Hyderabad**, Phone: Rel:+91-40-32940929, e-mail: hyderabad@jaypeebrothers.com
- **Kochi**, Phone: +91-484-2395740, e-mail: kochi@jaypeebrothers.com
- **Kolkata**, Phone: +91-33-22276415, e-mail: kolkata@jaypeebrothers.com
- **Lucknow**, Phone: +91-522-3040554, e-mail: lucknow@jaypeebrothers.com
- **Mumbai**, Phone: Rel: +91-22-32926896, e-mail: mumbai@jaypeebrothers.com
- **Nagpur**, Phone: Rel: +91-712-3245220, e-mail: nagpur@jaypeebrothers.com

***Overseas Offices***
- **North America Office, USA,** Ph: 001-636-6279734
  e-mail: jaypee@jaypeebrothers.com, anjulav@jaypeebrothers.com
- **Central America Office, Panama City, Panama**
  Ph: 001-507-317-0160, e-mail: cservice@jphmedical.com
  Website: www.jphmedical.com
- **Europe Office, UK,** Ph: +44 (0) 2031708910
  e-mail: info@jpmedpub.com

***Practical Management of Diabetes***


*First Edition:* **2010**

ISBN 978-81-8448-978-1

*Typeset at* JPBMP typesetting unit
*Printed at* Replika Press Pvt. Ltd.

# FOREWORD

Diabetes has assumed epidemic proportions the world over and India is the epicenter. India has the dubious distinction of being the world capital of diabetes.

Diabetes is a silent killer and a cause for a lot of morbidity and suffering. These days we find an earlier onset of diabetes in the population, which means that we need to treat these patients aggressively so that they can be complication free for many years to come.

The understanding of diabetes and treatment modalities have undergone a sea change in recent times. It is essential that all practicing doctor be updated with these advances so that they can do justice to their patients.

This book aims to do just that. Dr Ajit Kumthekar (my friend) is the right person for this job. His experience in managing diabetes is well known. Besides being a good clinician, he is actively involved in academics and is closely involved with the Research Society for the Study of Diabetes in India (RSSDI) as its joint secretary. Patient education has been an important area of focus for Dr Kumthekar. The innovations in patient management and treatment propounded by Dr Kumthekar are universally accepted.

This book is concise, to the point and informative, and packs all the information needed for a practicing doctor to upgrade his knowledge and skills in treating diabetes.

This book has Dr Kumthekar's trademark of simplicity, precision and authority written all over it.

**Vijay Panikar** MD MCPS FCPS DNB
Professor of Medicine
KJ Somaiya Medical College
Mumbai, Maharashtra, India

Consultant
Department of Endocrinology, Diabetes and Metabolism
Lilavati Hospital and Research Center
Mumbai, Maharashtra, India

# PREFACE

Modern medical science has controlled or eradicated many infectious diseases. A new set of diseases has started bothering human race for last few decades. These diseases are called life-style diseases. These include type II diabetes, hypertension, ischemic heart disease and malignancies. These have no curative treatment. If properly controlled, person with lifestyle disease can lead a near-normal life.

Type II diabetes is the result of insulin resistance and beta cell failure. Out of these two, beta cell failure is genetically determined while insulin resistance is mainly due to environmental factors with some genetic contribution. Lack of physical activity, increase in automation in all areas of life, disproportionately high calorie diet with low fiber content, rising use of nicotine and "stress" of modern age are the main factors which lead to insulin resistance.

The disease remains silent for a few years. The process of microvascular and macrovascular damage begins simultaneously. By the time the person becomes symptomatic, the complications have already set in. In fact, major vascular complication can be the presenting feature of this multiorgan disease.

The United Kingdom Prospective Diabetes Study (UKPDS) has shown that proper glucose control and blood pressure control slows down microvascular complications and offers some benefit to macrovascular complications too. The concept of glucose memory has emphasized the importance of good metabolic control during early years of this disease.

A Diabetes Outcome Progression Trial (ADOPT), Veterans Affairs Diabetes Trial (VADT), Action in Diabetes and Vascular Disease–Preterax and Diamicron Modified Release Controlled Evaluation (ADVANCE), DREAM, RECORD and BARI-2 are just to name the few trials which have guided the clinician as far as evidence-based decision-making is concerned. Action to Control Cardiovascular Risk in Diabetes (ACCORD) trial has cautioned us against too much aggression while managing diabetes with complications. It has identified a previously unrecognized harm of intensive glucose lowering in high-risk patients with type II diabetes.

A clinician needs a compact book in his office or the wards for ready-reference that will give up-to-date information in concise form. An attempt is being made to fulfill the need of thousands of primary care physicians who look after diabetic patients especially during initial phase of the disease. Various trials have proved the fact that if the patients get proper care during first 5 golden years of the illness, then the long-term benefits are immense.

I hope this book will provide necessary information for primary care physicians to provide good diabetes control of their patients.

I sincerely thank all those who have provided guidance and encouragement for writing this book. I must acknowledge the cooperation from my patients who have given me immense practical experience in management of this complex disease. I wish to offer my sincere thanks to Dr Vijay Panikar, Dr Vijay Neglur, Dr CS Yagnik and others who have been considered as icons in this field for their valuable suggestions. Support from my dietician Ms Vaihbhavi and my wife Shri Geeta is priceless. Last but not the least, I must thank the team of Jaypee Brothers Medical Publishers (P) Ltd especially Shri Jitendar P Vij (Chairman and Managing Director), Mr Ramesh Krishnan (Mumbai Branch) who have taken special efforts to print and publish this concise book on diabetes.

**Ajit B Kumthekar**

# CONTENTS

# ABBREVIATIONS

| | |
|---|---|
| ACEI | Angiotensin-converting enzyme inhibitor |
| AER | Albumin excretion rate |
| AGI | Alpha glucosidase inhibitor |
| ARB | Angiotensin receptor blocker |
| CCB | Calcium channel blockers |
| CHF | Congestive heart failure |
| DN | Diabetic nephropathy |
| DKA | Diabetic ketoacidosis |
| ESRD | End stage renal disease |
| GFR | Glomerular filtration rate |
| GIP | Glucose dependent insulinotropic polypeptide |
| GLP- 1 | Glucagon like peptide-1 |
| IGT | Impaired glucose tolerance |
| LSM | Lifestyle modification |
| SU | Sulfonylurea |
| OHA | Oral hypoglycemic agents |
| PCV | Packed cell volume |
| PP | Post-prandial |
| VPT | Vibration perception threshold |

# Chapter 1

# Introduction

Diabetes is defined as a metabolic disorder, which comes up due to absolute or relative deficiency of insulin.

Advances in medical science have been successful in reducing mortality and morbidity due to infectious diseases. There has been good success in controlling diseases related to undernutrition. But the new century in facing the problems of lifestyle diseases like ischemic heart disease, diabetes, hypertension and obesity. Prevalence of diabetes is on the rise and that too more so in developing countries.

As per the projection by WHO, India will be having highest number of diabetics in next few years.

| *Year →* / *Number* | *1994* | *2000* | *2010* |
|---|---|---|---|
| World prevalence | 98.3 | 157.3 | 215.6 |
| Number in Asia | 46.3 | 86.6 | 126.3 |
| Number in India | 20.0 | 35.0 | 55.0 |

- Numbers are in millions.

These figures take into account known diabetics. There are lot many undiagnosed diabetics and prediabetics in developing countries. The diabetes strikes at a relatively younger age, nearly a decade earlier as compared to western countries. This period of life is crucial for majority of people. They are working hard to achieve the targets of life, have lots of family responsibilities. Diagnosis of diabetes in mid-thirties is very likely to disturb their lifestyle and emotional set-up. Nicotine use is high in developing countries and alcohol use is on the rise due to modern wine-culture. Walking bare foot is not uncommon in these countries. Lack of adequate education, low economic status, difficult access to ideal health care facilities are some of the additional factors which need attention while managing these patients.

Rising cost of health care is also an important issue. Higher fees of doctors, more number of investigations, rising travel-costs and most important of all uncontrolled costs of majority of medications ... all of these result in higher expenditure for proper diabetes care. Although the cost of regular and thorough check-up is significantly less as compared to cost of treating complications, many patients are not able to get timely regular and complete check-up due to various reasons.

Comparative cost of diabetes care in India

| | |
|---|---|
| Yearly diabetic profile | 30 USD-1500 INR |
| Hemodialysis | 20 USD-1000 INR |
| Photocoagulation | 20 USD-1000 INR |
| Coronary angioplasty | 2,000 USD- 1,00,000 INR |
| CABG | 3,000 USD-1,50,000 INR |
| Foot amputation | 1,200 USD-60,000 INR |
| Renal transplantation | 2,000 USD-1,00,000 INR |

*Note*: These costs are representative of a semiurban set-up and may vary.

Patient and family members should be explained about these facts in order to have regular and completes check-up in future.

## PATHOPHYSIOLOGY OF DIABETES

- Type I diabetes is due to complete destruction of beta cells of islets of Langerhans in pancreas. The reason for this could be a viral infection or an autoimmune response. Some role HLA and genetic factors have been suggested.
- Type II diabetes is due to combination of three factors—Insulin resistance, incretin defect and beta cell deficiency. Insulin resistance is at the background. Incretin defect starts later and the ultimate event is beta cell dysfunction, which leads to deficiency of insulin.

Clinically, diabetes can be classified into following groups:

Type I diabetes, Type II diabetes, Gestational diabetes, Secondary diabetes.

Comparison of Type I and Type II diabetes

| *Type I* | *Type II* |
|---|---|
| Two percent of all diabetics | Ninety-eight percent % of all diabetics |
| Absolute insulin deficiency | Relative insulin deficiency |
| Age of onset below 20 years | Age of onset around 30 or above |
| Normal weight or underweight | Obese or high waist-hip ratio |
| Insulin is a must | Insulin may be needed |

### Gestational Diabetes

GDM is diagnosed when an abnormal glucose level is detected first time during pregnancy. The condition is more important for fetal growth and survival. Majority of these cases are managed by changes in diet and physical activity but some of them will need insulin to control high blood glucose.

Secondary diabetes is due to use of steroids, acromegaly, calcific pancreatitis, etc.

## NATURAL COURSE OF DIABETES

- Asymptomatic stage which may last for 3-5 years.
- Symptomatic stage.
- Stage of complications like nephropathy, cardiac involvement, neuropathy.
- Death.

In our clinical practice, we come across cases in asymptomatic stage or patients with minimal symptoms. When we advise about lifestyle change, minimal medication and regular follow-up, the usual answer from the patient is " I will try". After some years, we see the same patient with congestive heart failure or foot gangrene or impaired vision as a result of diabetic vasculopathy. He then urges us to do the best possible treatment. At that stage, our response is nothing more than "I will try!"

Diabetes has no curative treatment as on today. Once a diabetic, the patient is always a diabetic. Person has to follow dietary regulations and exercise even if his blood glucose level and other biochemical markers are within the normal limits. Clinician should explain to the patient that every attempt should be made to avoid complications by following advice offered by health care team. Basic diabetes care is provided by a team consisting of doctor, dietician, health educator and if possible an exercise trainer. A person with complications of diabetes will need a surgeon, cardiologist, nephrologist, an ophthalmologist and other specialists. The cost of diabetes care escalates rapidly once the complications set in. Moreover the complications come up one after another. A person with neuropathy will soon develop retinopathy or nephropathy. A person who undergoes leg amputation will have risk of getting acute coronary insufficiency. This again emphasizes the importance of avoiding complications at all costs.

## SEEKING FOR CURE

Many a times diabetic patients are misguided by some people, who suggest cure from diabetes. They offer some fancy or traditional medications with a heavy price tag. Many of them contain nephrotoxic compounds like heavy metals. There is always a risk in trying these unscientific means and our patients should be specifically warned against this. I have seen patients who got transient control of hyperglycemia with such medications but within few months these patients landed up with end stage renal disease. If a person wants to try out such medicines then he should do it at his own risk. Moreover he should be told to try only one system of medicine at a time, and not to combine them. No authentic information is available about drug interaction between herbal medicines and medicines from modern science. These points should be explained to the patient and relatives during first few meetings.

Chapter 2

# Taking History of a Diabetic Person

As diabetes is a silent disease in vast majority of patients, detailed information must be sought by in-depth history taking. Patient reaching your clinic might be a known diabetic for last many years or may be a freshly detected diabetic. Hence, a printed questionnaire in local language, covering all aspects of history, should be provided to every new diabetic person coming to your clinic for the first time for consultation. This method will ensure that no major point is missed out. Many a times people stop medication for months together, recent blood tests reports are not available. In such situations in particular, this method of history taking is very useful.

## HISTORY SHEET

1. Name Age Sex
2. Address
3. Contact information:
   Landline: Best time to contact:
   Cell phone: Best time to contact:
   E-mail address:
4. *Year of detection of diabetes*: Duration of diabetes.
5. Symptoms at the time of diagnosis:
   a.
   b.
   c.
   d.
6. Treatment taken at that time:
7. *Benefit out of treatment*: Total, partial, and nil or cannot decide.
8. Present complaints

9. Ask specifically for:
   *Cardiac complaints*: Chest pain, breathlessness, palpitations.
   *GI complaints*: Nausea, bloating, and retrosternal pain, constipation.
   *Neuropathy symptoms*: Tingling numbness, burning soles.
   *Sexual dysfunction*: Erectile dysfunction.
   *Visual problems*: Double vision, impaired vision.
   Symptoms indicative of hypoglycemia.
10. *Current medications*: Dosage and timing—in as much details as possible.
11. Recent blood reports if any.
12. *Family history of diabetes*: Parents, brothers-sisters, distant relatives.
13. *Exercise pattern of the patient*: Type, frequency, and regularity.
14. Dietary habits
    A. Daily diet

| *Breakfast* | *Rice-flakes* | *Bread* | *Cereals* | *Others* | |
|---|---|---|---|---|---|
| Lunch | Bread/chapatti | Rice | Vegetables | Pulses | Nonvegetarian item |
| Afternoon snacks | Tea | Bread | Biscuits | Other | |
| Dinner | Bread/chapatti | Rice | Vegetables | Pulses | Nonvegetarian item |

    B. Favorite food items.
    C. Consumption of oil per person in a month.
    D. Use of groundnuts, dry coconut or oil seeds.
    E. Use of artificial sweeteners.
    F. Do you consume fish/chicken/meat? If yes, then how frequently.

G. Do you use raw vegetables, salads or fruits regularly?
H. Do you sieve wheat flour?

15. *Addictions*: Tobacco in any form, alcohol, any other.
16. Whether complete work-up was done in past? Reports?
17. Do you have basic knowledge about diabetes?
18. Do you use any traditional or nonprescription medications?

Remember, proper history taking will make you familiar with your patient whom you are going to manage for rest of his life.

Chapter 3

# Diagnosis of Diabetes

Early and complete diagnosis is the 1st important step in managing diabetic patients.

The disease is silent for many years. High index of suspicion is needed to pick-up the cases before it is too late.

Clinical situations in which blood glucose estimation should be asked for:

- Classical symptoms – Polyuria, polydipsia, polyphagia
- Weight loss despite good or excessive appetite
- Recurrent infections – Skin or urinary tract or respiratory
- Tingling numbness in limbs
- All cases of IHD
- Hypertensive patient
- Person with renal impairment
- Lady with PCOD
- Lady who had recurrent abortions
- During antenatal check-up
- Lady who has delivered a large (Above 10 lb) baby
- Executive medical check-up
- Nonhealing wound
- Person with herpes zoster.
- Person with periarthritis of shoulder
- Person with tuberculosis
- Person with TIA or CVA
- Person with noncompressive 3rd cranial nerve or 6th cranial nerve palsy
- Blood relatives of diabetic person who are above 35 years of age
- Person having heel ache specifically at 1st step in morning
- Person with intermittent claudications

- At the time of medical insurance
- All overweight and obese people
- Those having central obesity
- Those who are addicted to tobacco and/or alcohol
- Those with raised triglycerides and low HDL
- Before any surgical procedure

Apart from this, in India one can come across a patient with diagnosis of diabetes when it is least suspected (i.e. a hardworking, normal weight farmer without any family history of diabetes is found to have diabetes during a diagnostic camp in his village!) Therefore, high index of suspicion is a must for early diagnosis.

## HOW TO CONFIRM CLINICAL SUSPICION?

Measurement of blood glucose is the only way to confirm diagnosis of diabetes. Measurement of HbA1C or checking urine for sugar is of no use for diagnosing diabetes. The former test is of some use to judge the duration of diabetes in a freshly detected hyperglycemic case, the later test does not provide any clinically relevant information, hence should not be done.

Recently, it is being suggested that HbA1C if above 6.5 % can be used as a diagnostic test for diabetes. But there is no unanimous agreement on this issue.

Minimum 8 hours of fasting is needed before a sample of venous blood is collected. 1 cc sample should be collected in fluoride bulb for estimating glucose. At this moment it is wise to collect blood (1cc in EDTA and 3 cc in plain bulb) so that we can perform tests included under "Diabetic profile" on the same day, in case the person is found to have diabetes. If possible, person should be instructed beforehand to bring

1st urine sample in any clean container when he comes for giving blood sample. This instruction is useful when one wants to perform micro-albuminuria test in a diabetic person. In case this instruction was not given or was not followed by the person, then one can ask for urine sample immediately after collecting fasting blood sample. This can be used to perform routine urine analysis with special attention to ketones, proteins, pus cells, etc.

Thereafter oral glucose challenge with 75 grams of glucose, dissolved in 200 ml of water, is offered to the person. Glucose water should be consumed gradually over 5-10 minutes in order to avoid nausea and vomiting. Exact Time at which glucose consumption was begun is to be noted. Precisely 120 minutes from that time, 1 cc of blood sample should be collected in fluoride bulb.

Diagnostic criteria

| | *Normal* | *Prediabetes* | *Diabetes* |
|---|---|---|---|
| Fasting | Below 100 mg% | 100-126 mg% | Above 126 mg % |
| 2 hr post-glucose | Below 140 mg% | 140-200 mg% | Above 200 mg% |

Once we that a person is diabetic by using these criteria, the next important step will be to assess the extent of target organ damage. The tests commonly done for this purpose are grouped together under the name of "Diabetic Profile".

These tests are:

- Lipid profile
- S. creatinine
- S. GPT (S. ALT)
- Hemoglobin and WBC count
- HbA1C
- Urine routine and for micro-albuminuria

- ECG
- Fundoscopy by an ophthalmologist
- VPT for peripheral neuropathy
- Vascular Doppler if PVD is suspected

Results of all the tests mentioned above will give you complete diagnosis of a diabetic person.

These tests help us in choosing the correct medication for a freshly detected diabetic. These tests warn us about possible side effects or dosage adjustment of oral anti-hyperglycemic agents, e.g. high S. creatinine will prevent you from using Metformin and high S. GPT will not allow you to use Glitazones. Presence of ketones in urine will justify the use of insulin at the onset, and proteinuria will demand ACE inhibitors in your prescription.

Similarly, dyslipidemia will need statins or fibrates, and abnormal baseline ECG will emphasize use of aspirin. HbA1C beyond 10 % will suggest the need for immediate insulin in order to have rapid control of hyperglycemia as no orally effective medication can lower HbA1C by more than 2% (Target of HbA1C is 7 %). Person with abnormal VPT should be given detailed information about foot care.

These tests should be performed at initial diagnosis and they should be repeated once a year. Some of these tests may be repeated more often in case the baseline reports are abnormal. Therefore, it is wise to collect fasting blood sample in all the 3 bulbs (plain bulb, fluoride bulb and EDTA bulb) in the morning.

For follow-up, fasting and 2 hrs postlunch blood samples are collected. For postmeal sample, time is measured from beginning of meal. If the patient is taking medication at breakfast then the routine should not be changed on the day of testing. After giving fasting blood sample he should take morning dose at breakfast, then have lunch approx. 3-4 hrs later. Blood sample should be collected 2 hrs after lunch and not 2 hrs after breakfast. This will maintain the proper pharmacokinetics of anti-diabetic medications on the day of testing and thus will reflect precise glycemic state on that day.

You have to look beyond blood sugar report when you are managing diabetic patients. You have to explain this concept to the patient and relatives so that clinical decision making becomes easier. Remember, you are not treating a piece of paper with blood sugar report on it but you are managing life of a human being with metabolic derangement. Therefore a complete diagnosis is a must at the beginning of this life-long journey.

Serum insulin level, C-peptide levels, testing for GAD or Islet cell antibodies are rarely needed for clinicians. They are mainly used as research tools.

### How to Interpret Test Results?

| *Name of the test* | *Normal range* |
|---|---|
| 1. Fasting blood glucose | 70-100 mg/dl |
| 2. 2 hrs post-glucose | 100-140 mg/dl |
| 3. S. cholesterol | < 200 mg /dl |
| 4. HDL | In men above 40 mg/dl<br>In women above 35 mg /dl |
| 5. LDL | < 100 mg/dl |
| 6. Triglyceride | < 150 mg/dl |
| 7. Hemoglobin | 11-14.5 gm/dl |
| 8. S. creatinine | < 1.4 mg/dl |
| 9. S. GPT | < 40 IU/L |
| 10. HbA1C | < 7 % |

*Contd...*

*Contd...*

| *Name of the test* | *Normal range* |
|---|---|
| 11. Micral | < 19 mg/L |
| 12. ECG | Normal |
| 13. VPT | < 15 volts |
| 14. Fundoscopy | No retinopathy |

If the patient has got hyperglycemia with all other tests within normal limits then he is said to be in safe zone. If at all one or two tests from diabetic profile are abnormal, then appropriate steps are taken to correct the metabolic abnormality. This is usually achieved with minimal number of drugs in lowest possible dosage.

This was in short about clinician's approach to a newly diagnosed diabetic patient.

---

As per latest information—ADA has included A1C > 6.5% as one of the diagnostic criteria as per clinical practice recommondations 2010.

Chapter 4

# Medical Nutrition in Diabetes

Knee jerk reaction to first abnormal blood glucose report of any diabetic patient is deleting rice, sugar, potatoes and fruits from his plate. Dietary guidelines offered to a diabetic person should be more scientific and precise. It should consider usual dietary habits in the community, daily routine of the individual, family income and festivals (e.g. Diwali, Ramadan or Christmas). Special care should be taken during marriage season too.

Ideal body weight of the person should be found out from the patient's height. BMI less than 25 and more than 19 is desirable. Depending upon his physical activity level, total daily caloric need is calculated. Food items that fulfill this caloric need should be chosen. There should be a good blend to provide necessary proteins, fats, minerals, vitamins, fiber and trace elements too.

Food intake should be in small portions and there should be at least two major meals, two snacks and one or two light refreshments. The concepts of exchange list, artificial sweeteners, and sick day schedule should be explained to patient and the family members. Selected fruits should be consumed daily. Low salt diet should be preferred over preserved food items containing large amount of sodium.

Not more than two days of fast are allowed per month.

Sample diet charts for 1200/ 1600/1800 calories to be used by diabetic patients and some interesting recipes are given in appendix.

For practical reasons I handover a table of food items from which a patient can choose or refuse food item for his meal or snacks. My dietician then informs about timing and quantity of food items that are allowed.

Dietary guideline chart

| *Allowed food items* | *Limited food items* | *Restricted food items* |
|---|---|---|
| Wheat, Soybean | Rice, Baajri | Sago, Sweets |
| Jowar, Nagli | Rice-flakes | Potato-chips |
| Curry | Popcorn, cornflakes | Chana daal- fried items |
| Skimmed milk, Yogurt | Milk with cream, Jam | Milk powder |
| Buttermilk, Soup | Fruit jelly, Fruit custard | Butter |
| Leafy vegetables | Brinjal, Pumpkin | Glucose, Honey, Jaggery |
| Sprouts | Green peas | Cheese |
| Guar, Karela | Potato with skin | Ice-cream |
| Onion, Tomato, Carrot | Fish, mutton | Broiler chicken |
| Ladies fingers | Cashew nuts, Almonds | Yellow of egg |
| Fresh coconut | Red chilies | Dry coconut |
| White of egg | Spices | Dates, Black pepper, Groundnuts |
| Papaya, watermelon | Oranges, Apple | Banana, Mango, Grapes |
| Figs, Sweet lime, Pomegranate, Pineapple | Guava, Cherries | Custard apple, Chikko, Dried fig |
| Marie biscuits | Bread slice | Fried food |
| Roasted pepped | Oily non-vegetarian item | Samosa |
| Dhokla | Mixed pickles | Cakes, Chocolates |
| Daliya, Idli | Sugar | Mango pickle |
| Coconut water | Limca, Thums-up | Mangola |
| Tea/coffee without sugar | Lime sorbet | Frozen food |
| Water from Daal | Bournvita, Horlicks | Fast food |

*Note*:
- Jaggery and groundnuts in curry and vegetables are allowed.
- Fenugreek seed help in reducing blood glucose.

Chapter 5

# Exercise for Diabetes

One of the important but often neglected feature of diabetes care is exercise. Doctors forget to give specific exercise prescription and patients come up all sorts of excuses for not doing regular exercise. Most of the exercise types that are recommended by a physician cost almost nothing as opposed to costly medications. Consistency, adequacy and proper combination of various exercise types are important aspects of exercise.

| *Positive effects of exercise* | *Risks of exercise* |
|---|---|
| Reduces blood sugar | Hypoglycemia |
| Reduces hyperinsulinemia | Hyperglycemia after intense exercise |
| Reduces insulin resistance | Ketoacidosis after intense exercise |
| Fall in glycated hemoglobin | Worsening of retinopathy |
| Reduces blood pressure | Aggravation of proteinuria |
| Improves pattern of lipid profile | Risk of foot injury |
| Improves body composition | Aggravation of IHD |
| Reduces cardiovascular risk | |
| Improves quality of life | |
| Gives more flexibility /stamina | |

Before you recommend any exercise to a diabetic person, it is better to screen for chronic complications of diabetes. Anyone with proliferative retinopathy or microalbuminuria or autonomic or peripheral neuropathy should be advised correct exercise that is less likely to aggravate these problems. Careful cardiac assessment should be carried out in older diabetics. TMT (CST) will give information about abnormal blood pressure response to exercise and silent ischemia in diabetics.

## TYPES OF EXERCISE

Types of exercise are:
- Aerobic
- Resistance
- Flexibility

Moderate intensity aerobic exercise lasting for 30 minutes is suitable for majority of patients. The most popular and easy to perform exercise is walking. It should be for minimum 30 minutes and above, and should be without a break. This can be achieved if person keeps slow or medium pace of walk. Continuous muscle activity for more than 30 minutes results in burning of body fat while short bursts of high intensity exercise consumes glucose. Recommended total duration of aerobic exercise is 150 minutes per week.

Exercise session should begin with warming up for 5 minutes and should end by relaxation or cooling down for 5 minutes. Main portion of exercise should be moderate intensity. It should last for 30 minutes. Target heart rate achieved should be 50 to 70% of maximal heart rate for the patient. Maximal heart rate is calculated by subtracting age in years from 220.

*For Example*

Maximal heart rate for a person aged 50 years is 170.

Target heart rate say 60% would be 102 beats per minute

Aerobic exercise that maintains this heart rate for 30 minutes would be adequate to provide cardiovascular benefits.

Suggested walking schedule for beginners

| | Time (minutes) | | | |
|---|---|---|---|---|
| *Weeks* | *Warming up* | *Brisk walk* | *Cooling down* | *Total* |
| 1 | 5 | 5 | 5 | 15 |
| 2 | 5 | 10 | 5 | 20 |
| 3 | 5 | 15 | 5 | 25 |
| 4 | 5 | 20 | 5 | 30 |
| 5 | 5 | 25 | 5 | 35 |
| 6 | 5 | 30 | 5 | 40 |

Resistance exercises should not be more than 10% of total exercise. It should include all major muscle groups. Weights used should be light during initial period. Three sets of 8-10 repetitions of each muscle groups are usually adequate. Resistance exercises should be performed 2-3 times a week.

Flexibility exercises include stretching and Yoga. They are useful in providing normal muscle tone. They help in relaxation of body and soul! Yoga can be considered as an ad-on exercise towards basic aerobic exercise, something like main income and side-income. Person is free to practice Yoga provided he has time and energy after doing aerobic exercise.

## TIMING OF EXERCISE

The patient should decide the timing of exercise that he can follow regularly for days after days. One should not perform heavy exercise immediately after major meal. Timing of peak action of medication (especially insulin and SU) should not coincide with peak of exercise.

Usually, early morning exercise is preferred timing of exercise for majority of diabetics.

## FREQUENCY OF EXERCISE

Aerobic exercise—3-5 times a week.

Gap between exercise—days should not be more than 2 days as the effect of exercise on insulin resistance weans off after 48 hours.

Resistance exercise should be done 2-3 times per week.

Special precautions and suggestions for patient with diabetic complication

| *Complication* | *Discouraged activity that involves* | *Suggested activity that involves* |
|---|---|---|
| Severe NPDR or PDR | Valsalva's maneuver, jarring or pounding | Low impact exercises |
| Peripheral neuropathy | Repetitive stepping | Nonweight bearing exercises |
| Autonomic neuropathy | Unsupervised high intensity exercise | Low intensity, non-repetitive, slower pace |

Following points should be considered while writing a exercise prescription:

- Expectations of the patient and family members
- Establishing realistic goals
- Type of suitable exercise for the particular patient
- Timing of medication and food
- Appropriate footwear
- Checking blood sugar especially in type I cases
- Management of hypoglycemia
- Frequency, duration and intensity of exercise
- Rate of progression of exercise
- Monitoring results.

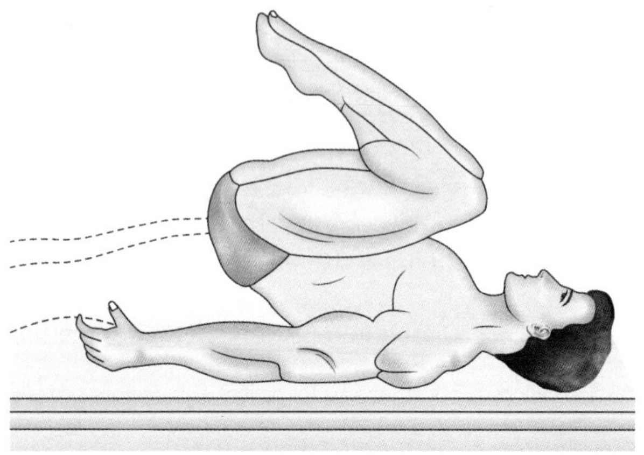

**Figure 5.1:** Back rolling

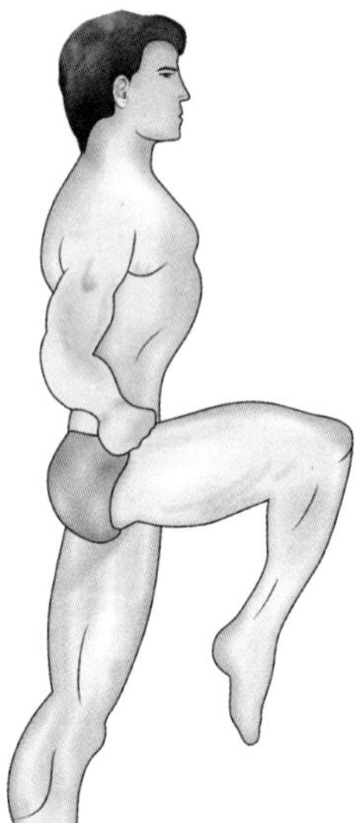

**Figure 5.2:** Spot jogging

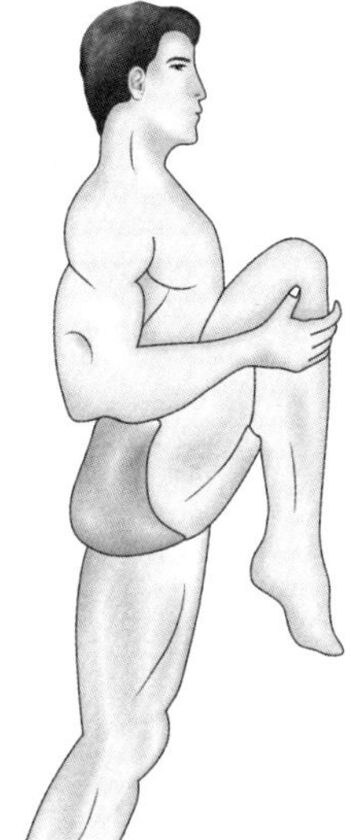

**Figure 5.3:** Knee-chest position-I

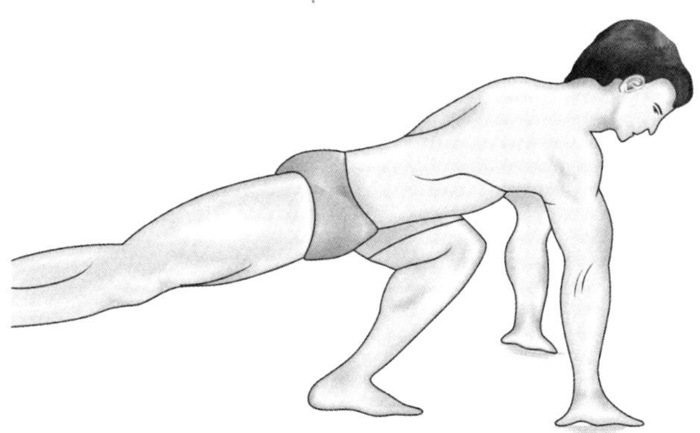

**Figure 5.4:** Knee-chest position-II

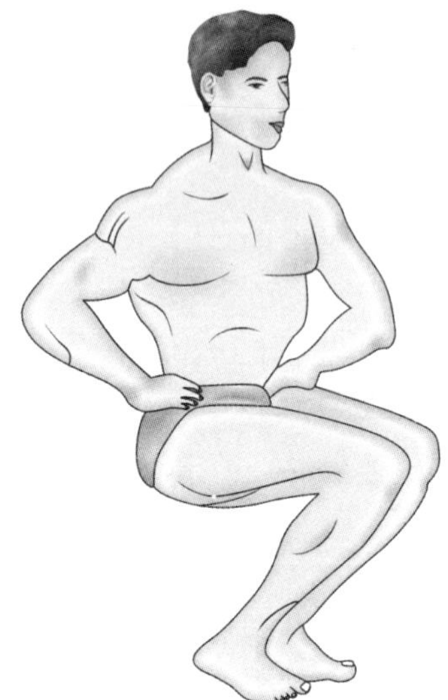

**Figure 5.5:** Squats

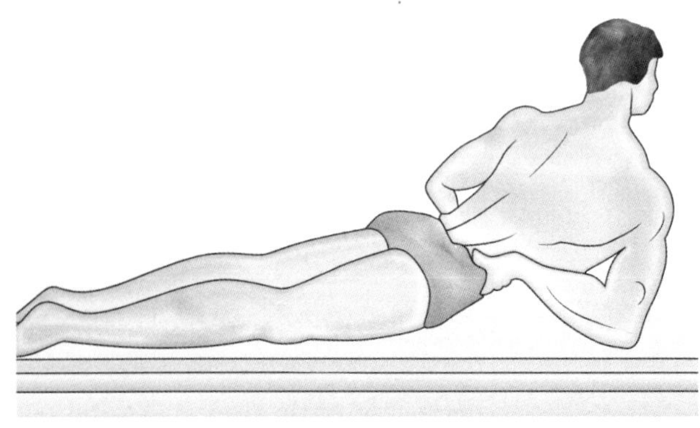

**Figure 5.6:** Back stretching-I

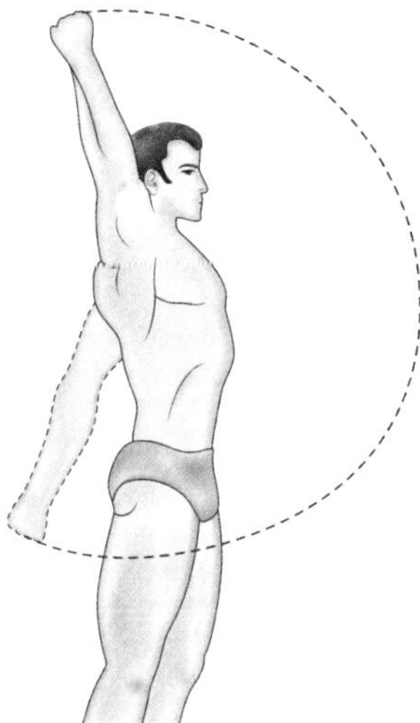

**Figure 5.7:** Back stretching-II

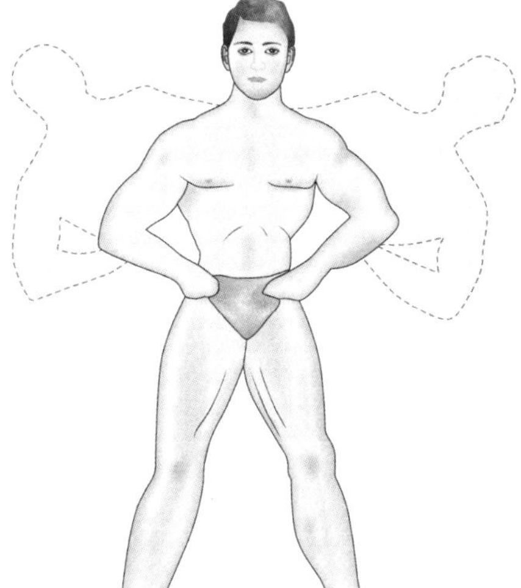

**Figure 5.8:** Side-swings

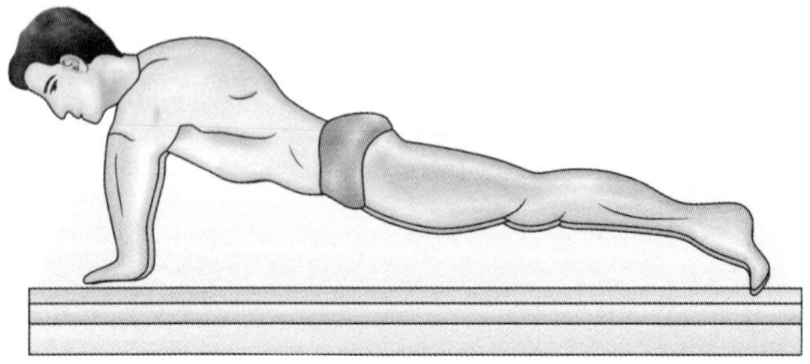

**Figure 5.9:** Push-ups

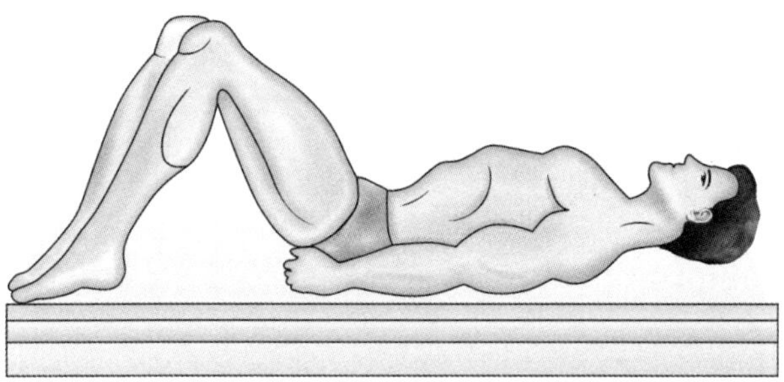

**Figure 5.10:** Relaxing at the end

Many physicians do not discuss exercise as modality of treatment with diabetic patients. The reason could be either lack of time or lack specific knowledge about exercise prescription. He is missing an opportunity use this means of controlling metabolic derangement in the patient. As a responsible physician, one should make a sincere attempt to motivate every diabetic patient to begin with simple exercise-patterns and move on steadily so that it becomes a part of their lifestyle. Regular exercise provides good glucose control, remarkable weight loss, reduces cardiac risk and offers a sense of well-being—in short it improves quality of life. That is the only thing everyone is asking for.

Chapter 6

# Education in Diabetes

As on today there is no cure for diabetes. We can achieve good control of diabetes by lifestyle modification (Diet, exercise and de-addiction) with proper use of medications. These means are more effective if adequate education of the diabetic person and his family members is carried out. In addition to this, there is a need for educating the society in general about this rapidly spreading disease.

A diabetic person is emotionally disturbed when the diagnosis of diabetes is declared to him. He tries to seek information and suggestions from all directions and becomes more confused. Some guidelines form relatives and friends are misleading and scientifically incorrect. What he needs is proper scientific information in simple language, which will boost his confidence. I tell my patients that God has given you an opportunity to pay attention to your body. Consider diabetes as a second inning in which you can correct your mistakes and score a century! This gives some confidence to the newly diagnosed diabetic patient.

## EDUCATION OF THE PATIENT

### Nature of the Illness

- Importance of good control of diabetes:
- Concept of diabetic profile—Look beyond blood sugar
- Need for regular monitoring.

### Myths and Realities about Diet

- Concept of glycemic index, carbohydrate counting and exchange list.
- N6–N3 ration of various edible oils.

- Class I proteins for patient with proteinuria.
- Fear about fruits.

### Exercise Benefits

Mixing of various exercise patterns – Aerobic, resistance and stretching.

- Motivation for regular workout
- Choice of in-door exercise, especially for women.
- Avoiding foot injury for patient with neuropathy.

### De-addiction

- Explain link between tobacco and atherosclerosis.
- Burst the myth of cardioprotective effects of alcohol.
- Inform that erectile dysfunction is common in alcoholics.
- Discuss about de-addiction options.

### Oral Hypoglycemic Agents

- Explain the mode of action of chosen agent, in simple language.
- Insist on proper timing of taking tablets (Before, with or after food).
- Inform about common side effects (SU-hypo, AGI-bloating).
- Discuss limitations of oral hypoglycemic agents.
- Reduce dose or hold them for a day of two when food intake is low.
- Explain inherent risks of herbal medications—nephropathy.

### Use of Other Medications in a Diabetic

- Avoid liquid medications with syrupy base.
- Avoid steroids, thiazide diuretics.
- Safety of sweeteners.

### Insulin

- Wipe out misconceptions and fears about insulin.
- Inform about newer delivery devices and newer insulins.
- Explain about proper storage of insulin.
- Proper timing of insulin injection.
- Correct technique and syringe for injecting insulin.

### Hypoglycemia

- Clinical situation at which hypo can occur.
- Important symptoms of hypo.
- Timely primary care.
- Carrying ID and sugar cubes.

### Complications of Diabetes

- Silent for many years since the onset.
- Can be detected by simple test like ECG, microalbuminuria, VPT, and fundoscopy if done regularly.
- Progression can be slowed down with medication.
- Commonly used proverb that can be used to educate diabetes—A stitch in time saves nine!

### Foot Care

- Especially important for rural population who walk barefoot.

- Daily foot care and examination.
- Proper cutting of nails.
- Ideal footwear.
- Early and proper care of minor wounds and ulcers.
- Paying attention to change in color of foot.

## EDUCATION OF FAMILY MEMBERS AND FRIENDS

- Encourage patient to follow dietary guidelines and exercise schedule.
- Help to follow proper instructions about medicines.
- Help him to quit nicotine use and alcohol addiction.
- Help a very young type I diabetic to take insulin.
- Financial support for medical care.
- Avoid marriage between two families having strong history of diabetes.

## EDUCATION OF SOCIETY MEMBERS

- Healthy food habits for the society in general.
- Promotion of active lifestyle.
- Less of automation wherever possible.
- Awareness about hazards of nicotine and alcohol.
- Concept of ideal body weight and ideal body composition.
- Stress management.

## MEANS TO PROVIDE EDUCATION ABOUT DIABETES

- Verbal-during consultation at clinic.
- Printed material providing basic information about disease.

- Audiocassettes or audio CD for illiterates.
- DVD or VCD for home viewing.
- Audiovisual presentation.
- Group discussion or question-answer sessions.
- Drama or a short documentary or a puppet show in villages.
- Internet—explain the risks of getting too much of knowledge!

If we succeed in educating masses about diabetes, then we may slow down the spread of this deadly epidemic in the world. United efforts of medical professionals, social workers, stage artists, government agencies, spiritual and religious leaders will offer some fruitful results.

Chapter 7

# Pharmacotherapy of Type II Diabetes

Today's physician is fortunate enough to have multiple agents at his disposal to control hyperglycemia. There are 5 types of oral -hypoglycemic agents – (OHA) -SU, Metformin, AGI, TZD and DPP-IV inhibitors available. These agents reduce blood glucose by different modes of action. SU and DPP-IV inhibitors are insulin secretogogues. Metformin and TZD act by reducing insulin resistance. AGI slows down rate of breakdown of complex carbohydrates in intestine by competitive inhibition of enzymes in intestinal wall. Therefore, the actions of these drugs, when combined, are complementary to each other.

Following discussion is focused on well-established means for controlling hyperglycemia in type II diabetic patient. Newer molecules like exanatide, liraglutide, sitagliptine and vildagliptin (Incretin based therapies) are discussed in a separate chapter of this book.

*Newly detected type II diabetic is either*:
*Mild*: Fasting BSL- (F BSL) < 130 mg %,
*Moderate*: F BSL 130- 270 mg %, A1C < 10%
*Severe*: F BSL above 270 mg % and A1C above 10%.

## MILD TYPE II DIABETIC PERSON

Mild type II diabetic person is advised to follow lifestyle modification (LSM), i.e. diet, exercise and de-addiction. Blood sugar is monitored every 2-3 months. Oral hypoglycemic agent is added if blood sugar is not adequately controlled with lifestyle modification. Initial drug of choice is either metformin or TZD or AGI in these patients.

## MODERATE TYPE II DIABETICS

Moderate type II diabetics are given OHA along with LSM from the beginning of therapy. If the person has features of insulin resistance (Obesity, acanthosis nigricans, hypertension, dyslipidemia) then the choice of 1st drug is Metformin. On the other hand if he has features of insulin deficiency (underweight, profound symptoms) then the 1st drug is SU. It is quite common observation that most of the diabetics are not adequately controlled with use of single OHA. Combination of agents from 2 groups is a must in most of the cases and agents from 3 groups is not uncommon, although the later has not been validated by randomized control trials.

Combination of SU and Metformin is the most popular, economical and effective combination of OHA. Combining short acting agent like glipizide or gliclazide with metformin will reduce risk of hypoglycemia. Combination of two insulin sensitizers – metformin and TZD—is useful as they act at different sites. Metformin or TZD can be combined with AGI when post-prandial hyperglycemia is the main issue. The latest oral agent- Sitagliptin–has been successfully combined with Metformin.

Combination of OHA is effective as long as there is some intrinsic insulin secretion. Gradually insulin secretion drops and so does the efficacy of combination of drugs. At this stage the patient has to be given exogenous insulin.

Effect of OHA combination on A1C and weight

| | *A1C change % against 1st agent alone* | *Weight change in kg against 1st agent alone* |
|---|---|---|
| Met added to SU | −1.0 | − 0 |
| TZD added to SU | −1.0 | Increase |
| TZD added to Metformin | −0.6 | Increase |
| SU added to Metformin | −1.0 | 2.0 |
| Sitagliptin + Metformin | −0.7 | – |

Even after initiating insulin therapy, OHA can be continued. Metformin and TZD improve insulin sensitivity to endogenous and exogenous insulin. It helps in reducing the dose of exogenous insulin. AGI reduce the rate of rise in postprandial blood glucose and thus offset the defect in 1st phase of insulin secretion seen in type II diabetics. SU when combined with exogenous insulin offer more physiological insulin response. It thus reduces chances of hypoglycemia.

Insulin with OHA – Effects on A1C and weight

| | *A1C % change versus prior treatment* | *Weight change in kg versus prior therapy* |
|---|---|---|
| Basal insulin to Met. | −2.5 | + 0.4 |
| Basal insulin to SU | −2.1 | + 2.0 |
| Basal insulin to SU + Met. | −1.9 | +1.2 |
| Met. added to insulin | −1.9 | −0.4 |
| SU + Insulin | −1.4 | +1.2 |
| TZD + Insulin | −1.3 | + 3.4 |
| AGI + Insulin | −0.6 | 0 |

Hypoglycemia is common with combination of SU and insulin. It is less common with Metformin and TZD.

Problems with TZD are slow onset of action and fluid retention, which is especially common with Rosiglitazone.

Best way to begin insulin in a patient who is inadequately controlled with oral agents is to give basal insulin (NPH or Glargine) 10 U at bedtime. F blood sugar is monitored every week. Depending upon F BSL, dose of basal insulin is adjusted.

This plan helps in achieving smooth control of fasting blood sugar with one injection per day. Postprandial excursions are managed by OHA.

Dose of basal insulin as per fasting blood glucose

| *F BSL* | *Dose of basal insulin* |
|---|---|
| 100 mg/dl | 10 U |
| 100-120 mg/dl | 12 U |
| 120-140 mg/dl | 14 U |
| 140-180 mg/dl | 16 U |
| Above 180 mg/dl | 18 U |

When F BSL is above 180 mg/dl, then the patient is no longer suitable for once a day insulin therapy. He needs either split mix insulin regimen or multiple daily insulin injections as in type I diabetics.

## SEVERE TYPE II DIABETICS

Severe type II diabetics with high F BSL and A1C require insulin in heavy dose (> 100 U/day), as they are insulin resistant. Insulin regimen is chosen as per the patient's glucose profile. One may need one injection of premixed insulin at breakfast, one injection of short acting insulin before lunch and one injection of premixed insulin before dinner. Basal insulin at bedtime and short acting insulin before each meal may be the need of some patients. Small number of cases are satisfactorily controlled with 2 injection of premixed insulin – one at breakfast and another at dinner. These cases can be given Metformin or TZD to have tight glucose control.

## PEARLS FOR DAY-TO-DAY PRACTICE

- When one OHA is not effective in controlling blood glucose, shifting to other OHA will not yield results. It is better to combine the agents form two groups to get desired results.
- Full therapeutic dose is not needed to achieve desired effect. Half of the maximal recommended dose is sufficient to know the efficacy of the drug.
- Adding third drug is not a scientifically proven approach. But many physicians do use this approach, as the patients are reluctant to start insulin.
- Basal insulin at night and OHA during day is as effective as multiple insulin dosage in early stage of severe type II diabetics in whom oral agents have failed.
- Multiple daily insulin injections are usually needed in advanced type II diabetics to achieve normal glucose level.
- Combine OHA from different groups will reduce incidence of adverse effects.
- Insulin levels, C-peptide measurements are rarely needed before starting insulin therapy.
- Small percentage of type II diabetics who are lean could be LADA (Late Onset Auto-immune Diabetes in Adult). They need insulin for glucose control within few years of

diagnosis. The condition can be detected by testing for GAD (Glutamic acid decarboxylase) antibodies.

- Concept of combining three drugs at the beginning of treatment is catching support from many clinicians.

Chapter 8

# Overview of Hypoglycemic Agents

It has been shown beyond doubt that morbidity and mortality due to diabetes is reduced by good control of blood sugar. Although multiple drugs are available to control hyperglycemia, only a small percentage of diabetic population achieves the desired target of HbA1C of 7 %.

The reasons for this situation are multiple. Being a silent disease the patient does not approach a doctor or does not follow the instructions correctly during the initial vital phase of the disease. As the nature of the disease is progressive, drug failure is the rule in most of the cases. Team approach to provide adequate education to the patient is not available at all places. Firm implementation of right intervention is not possible in many cases because of social, cultural and economic reasons. Diabetes supplies are not reimbursed by majority of insurance companies. Most of the therapy of a diabetic person is carried out as an out-patient (office based) case. The cost of such outpatient or office based treatment is not reimbursed by insurance people. Same is the problem about preventive measures. There are some unmet needs as far as therapeutic tools are considered. All the factors result in low adherence to treatment plans.

Depending upon our understanding of pathosphysiology of diabetes, various modalities of treatment are available. Type 1 diabetes is the result of absolute deficiency of insulin, hence insulin replacement is the only treatment used.

Type II diabetes is more complex. Insulin resistance, beta cell dysfunction and incretin defect are the three major factors in causation of this ailment. Glitazones and metformin reduce insulin resistance. Sulfonylureas (SU) and glinide group of drugs improve insulin secretion. Alpha-glucosidase inhibitor (AGI) reduces absorption of glucose from intestinal tract. Insulin replacement could be either basal or prandial depending upon severity of insulin deficiency. Incretin mimetics (Exanatide, liraglutide, taspoglutide) and incretin enhancers (Sitagliptin, vildagliptin, alogliptin, saxagliptin) correct the incretin defect found in Type II diabetes.

Various hypoglycemic or antihyperglycemic agents available

| | |
|---|---|
| Agents that reduce insulin resistance | Metformin, pioglitazone, rosiglitazone |
| Agents that induce insulin secretion | Sulfonylurea, glinides |
| Agents that reduce absorption of glucose from intestines | Acarbose, miglitol, voglibose |
| Insulin replacement | Basal or prandial insulin |
| Incretin based agents | Exenatide, liraglutide sitagliptin, vildagliptin |

Individual drugs from each group will be discussed in subsequent chapters. Basic information about the drugs is given in this chapter.

## DRUGS TO REDUCE INSULIN RESISTANCE

- Thiozolidinediones (Glitazones)
- Metformin

Glitazones (Rosiglitazone and pioglitazone) reduce insulin resistance at muscle, liver and fat cells. It results in decrease in hepatic glucose output and improvement in peripheral uptake of glucose. They reduce hepatic and visceral fat. These drugs act by binding with nuclear receptors (PPAR gamma), which regulate gene expression at transcription level. They are not effective in absence of insulin.

These drugs reduce blood glucose levels and show improvement in hyperinsulinemia. They have got some lipid lowering and antihypertensive effects too. Major side effects of these drugs are fluid retention. Hence, they are not advisable in patients with CCF. Slightly high incidence of humerus fractures has been reported with rosiglitazone.

Metformin is a good old drug, which was on back-foot for so many years because of unjustified fear of lactic acidosis. Recent therapeutic guidelines from Europe and USA have recommended metformin as a first drug after lifestyle modification. Exact mode of action of metformin is not clearly known. But reduction in hepatic glucose output and increasing GLP-1 levels are the two main pathways through which the drug exerts its anti-hyperglycemic effect. It has got some effect on lipids and blood pressure too. It can cause some reduction in body-weight.

This is the only drug that has shown improvement in macrovascular events in UKPDS study. It has also found to be effective in diabetes prevention trial. Through activation of AMPK, it may reduce cancer risk.

It does not cause hypoglycemia when used alone. Primary failure is uncommon and secondary failure is seen in about 30% cases. Side effects are mainly related to GI system and are mild and selflimiting. The drug is contraindicated in cases with CCF, hepatic failure and renal failure. Lactic acidosis is very rare if this drug is used judiciously.

## DRUGS THAT INCREASE INSULIN SECRETION

- Sulfonylurea group (SU)—Glipizide, glibenclamide (Glyburide), gliclazide, glimepiride.
- Glinide group—Repaglinide and nateglinide.

Sulfonylurea drugs act by stimulating beta cells of pancreas. Their effect is seen immediately after initiation of therapy. Hence, they provide quick symptomatic relief to diabetic patient. The medication should be taken 20-30 minutes before food intake. They can cause hypoglycemia and weight-gain. At times hypoglycemia can be protracted especially when the patient is on glibenclamide (Gliburide), or if the patient has consumed alcohol or there is renal/ hepatic failure. These drugs have no effect on lipids, blood pressure and cardiovascular risk.

Primary failure is seen in about 15% of cases and secondary failure rate is about 30%. Cost of therapy is low with these drugs.

Glinide group of drugs act by increasing insulin secretion. They have got short duration of action. These drugs are mainly effective to control postprandial hyperglycemia. Onset of action is fast and duration of action is short. The drug has to be taken just before food intake. Hypoglycemia is uncommon and mild. They are lipid neutral. Some weight gain is seen with these drugs. Overall cost of therapy is high with glinides.

## DRUGS WHICH REDUCE GLUCOSE ABSORPTION FROM GI TRACT

Alpha glucosidase inhibitor—Acarbose, miglitol, voglibose. These drugs block the activity of enzyme—Alpha glucosidase, thus, slowing the process of breaking down complex carbohydrates to simple sugars. These agents are to be taken at the first bite of food or during the meal. Main side effects are flatulence, diarrhea, rise in liver enzymes. They have shown some benefit in reducing CV risk in pre-diabetic patients.

## INSULIN REPLACEMENT

- Basal
- Prandial

All type I diabetics need insulin 3-4 times a day to have near normal glycemia. But in practice majority are on 2-3 injections per day.

In type II diabetics, as the years pass by beta cells no longer produce adequate insulin despite maximum dose of oral hypoglycemic agents. At this stage insulin is initiated. Usually, one begins with long acting insulin given at night-time (Basal supplementation) along with oral hypoglycemic agents during daytime. Later on as the insulin deficiency worsens the patient will need prandial insulin supplementation too.

## INCRETIN BASED THERAPIES

- Exenatide and liraglutide (Incretin mimetics).
- Sitagliptin and vildagliptin (DPP IV inhibitors).

Exenatide and liraglutide are in injectable form. Exenatide has short duration of action. Hence, the main benefit is control of postprandial hyperglycemia. As its action diminishes after 8-10 hours, it has got no effect on fasting hyperglycemia. It is to be given 30-60 minutes before meal. It has to be given twice daily. Usual dose is 5-10 mcg.

Sitagliptin and vildagliptin are in oral form.

Sitagliptin and vildagliptin are available DPP-IV inhibitors today. These molecules inhibit action DPP-IV thereby elevate GLP-1 and GIP. Inhibition is prolonged 12-24 hours. These agents reduce both fasting and PP hyperglycemia. Reduction in HbA1C is about 0.7 %. Usual dose of sitagliptin is 100 mg once daily and that of vildagliptin is 50 mg twice daily. Incase of renal impairment the dose of sitagliptin is reduced.

Diabetic patient of current generation is fortunate to have multiple agents that can be used to control blood sugar and other metabolic derangements. Judicious use these agents in rational combinations will prevent target organ damage. Combination will ensure that the dose of individual agent is submaximal. This will lower the chances of adverse effects of individual agents.

The latest suggestion of combining these agents at the beginning of diabetes is gaining popularity. Diabetes is the result of three pathophysiological processes—Insulin resistance, beta cell dysfunction and incretin defect. The disease remains silent for 5-8 years before it is diagnosed. There is evidence of macro- or microvascular damage at diagnosis in many patients.

The older concept of step care that involves adding one oral agent at each step does not achieve good control. The patient continues to have HbA1C above 8% for many years before he is shifted to insulin therapy. The vital period for good glucose control during first five years is lost. Hence, the concept of early combination therapy from the beginning of disease management is getting more and more popularity. Once good and stable control is achieved, one can lower the dosage and number of agents. In other words this too is a step care therapy (in different direction!).

# Chapter 9

# Sulfonylureas

The most commonly used oral hypoglycemic agent is from the group of drugs called sulfonylurea. These agents are very potent. They give quick clinical results and relatively inexpensive, hence, very popular amongst the patients and doctors. Nearly, 2/3rd of diabetic population have been given these drugs as initial treatment.

First generation sulfonylurea (SU) drugs were chlorpropamide, acetohexamide, tolbutamide. These agents are now replaced by second generation SU like glipizide, glibenclamide (Glyburide), gliclazide and glimepiride. Second generation SU have high intrinsic activity and potency due to higher affinity to binding sites on beta cells of pancreas.

## MECHANISM OF ACTION OF SULFONYLUREA

These agents act by closing ATP dependent potassium channels present on cell wall of beta cells. This action reduces membrane potential and opens calcium channels. Calcium moves from extracellular space to intracellular space. High calcium concentration leads to exocytosis of beta cell granules and insulin secretion.

There are some extrapancreatic effects of these agents.

- Potentiate insulin action
- Decrease in gluconeogenesis
- Step up hepatic glycogen synthesis.
- Inhibition of insuinase.

Many controversies exist about extrapancreatic actions of SU.

## CLINICAL EFFECTS OF SULFONYLUREA

These drugs mainly act by lowering fasting plasma glucose levels. They have some impact on early postprandial glycemic excursion but they have good effect on late postprandial rise in plasma glucose. As compared to placebo, these agents reduce HbA1C by 1.0 to 1.8% within 4 months.

Recently, diagnosed type II diabetic patient with fasting plasma glucose below 220 mg%, who is normal weight or slightly obese and one who has got good beta cell reserve (high C peptide level) is the best candidate for SU along with lifestyle modification.

UKPDS has shown that efficacy-wise they are comparable with insulin and have comparatively less chance of weight gain. The study has shown that these drugs show improvement in beta cell function by 78% but this improvement is not sustained over a period of time. At the end of 6 years, improvement in beta cell function is 52%.

Primary failure (no response after initiation of SU) is noted in patients with high fasting plasma glucose and low beta cell reserve. Secondary failure (gradual drop in responsiveness to SU) is seen in nearly 30% of cases.

All SU agents except glibenclamide are absorbed rapidly and completely after oral administration. Glibenclamide is slowly and incompletely absorbed. Micronized form of this agent is marginally better as far as rate and degree of drug absorption is concerned. Hyperglycemia delays absorption of these agents. Hence, they are more effective if given 30 minutes prior to food than when they are given with food.

These drugs are highly protein bound. They excreted in urine after metabolism.

Glipizide extended release tablet is available. This formulation provides steady drug level for nearly 24 hrs. Dose of such preparation 5-20 mg once daily.

Freshly detected, middle aged Type II diabetic should receive either a short acting SU if postprandial glucose level is high, or long acting SU if fasting hyperglycemia is the main problem. Short acting SU agents have inactive metabolites. Therefore, older people should receive these agents, as it will reduce the chances of getting hypoglycemia. Patients with renal impairment should be treated with short acting SU.

The debate over ischemic preconditioning has not come up with any definitive answer. As a clinician it would be wise to avoid glibenclamide in patients with underlying ischemic heart disease.

Persistent high concentrations of SU inhibit proinsulin biosynthesis and reduce insulin secretion. As against that discontinuous exposure of beta cells to SU is useful in maintaining acute insulin release. This is achieved by low dose once daily glipizide treatment.

SU failure could be either primary in 10-20% of cases. The cause of primary failure is marked insulin deficiency. Further 20-30% cases show secondary failure due to progressive loss of beta cells, lack of optimum lifestyle modification, desensitization after chronic exposure to SU.

Comparison of various sulfonylurea drugs

| *Name* | *Absorption* | *Half life* | *Metabolite* | *Dose* | *Note* | *Remark* |
|---|---|---|---|---|---|---|
| Glipizide | Rapid, complete | 1-5 hrs | Inactive | 2.5-10 mg | Improves acute insulin response | Safe, inexpensive |
| Gliclazide | Rapid, partial | 6-15 hrs | Inactive | 40-320 mg | Reduce platelet aggregation | Low-risk of weight gain and hypo |
| Glimepiride | Rapid, complete | 5-9 hrs | Active | 1-8 mg | 1st phase insulin secretion | Extrapancreatic actions No blocking of ischemic preconditioning |
| Glibenclamide | Slow, partial | 15-20 hrs | Active | 2.5-20 mg | Risk of hypo$^{++}$ | Potent, Inexpensive |

## COMBINATION OF SU WITH OTHER AGENTS

Combination of SU with other hypoglycemic agents is extremely effective. Best combination is SU$^{+}$ metformin. Other drugs like glitazones, alpha glucosidase inhibitors and insulin. By combining these drugs, dosage of individual drugs are reduced.

### Side Effects of Sulfonylurea

- Hypoglycemia—most commonly with glibenclamide.
- Weight gain—Approx. 2-3 kg.
- Lack of ischemic preconditioning. Not significant with usual dosage.
- Skin rashes.
- Drug interactions with alcohol, aspirin.

## CONTRAINDICATIONS OF SULFONYLUREA

- Pregnancy
- Type I diabetic
- Metabolic stress—Trauma, infection, infarct

- H/O skin allergy
- Advanced liver and renal disease.

## SUMMARY

- Potent and inexpensive drugs.
- Useful in early phase of disease.
- Can be easily combined with other agents.
- Long acting SU carry high-risk of hypoglycemia.
- Issue of ischemic preconditioning needs to be resolved.

# Chapter 10

# Meglitinides

Sulfonylureas (SU) are very potent drugs, which reduce blood sugar. But some of the limitations of these very popular drugs are risk of hypoglycemia, lack of flexibility for patient and inefficient control of post-prandial hyperglycemia. This led to invention of new class of anti-hyperglycemic agents called Meglitinides or Glinides in short.

These drugs differ from SU in chemical structure and pharmacokinetics. Repaglinide and nateglinides are two commonly used molecules from this group. Repaglinide is derived from meglitinede portion of SU and nateglinide is derived from amino acids. The third drug–Mitiglinide is still in investigational stage.

These drugs improve 1st phase of insulin release and thus have better effect on prandial glucose excursions. They are fast acting and their duration of action is short as compared to SU. They bind to specific site of SU receptor on beta cells and act via potassium dependent ATP channels.

## REPAGLINIDE

Repaglinide is 5 times more potent than glibenclamide. The action of repaglinide is glucose dependent. Repaglinide does not stimulate insulin secretion when there is complete lack of glucose. The best action of this drug is seen when the glucose concentration is in intermediate range.

Repaglinide is rapidly absorbed. Fat content of meal reduces degree of absorption. The peak plasma level is reached within 30 minutes. Elimination half-life is about 60 minutes. It is highly protein bound. The drug is degraded in liver cytochrome P450 enzyme. Main route of excretion is through bile and only 6% comes down in urine.

## NATEGLINIDE

Nateglinide is rapidly absorbed and its half-life is 1.5 hr. Only 10% of the drug is metabolized and is excreted in urine.

These agents can be used as monotherapy or in combination with metformin, glitazones or insulin. They can be used in age group of 18 to 75 years. Dose of repaglinide is 0.5 to 4 mg with each meal, and the maximum dose is 16 mg per day. Nateglinide is used in dose of 60 mg with each meal, the maximum dose is 180 mg/day. These agents are to be given just before meal or within 30 minutes of the meal.

## SAFETY OF MEGLITINIDES

As these drugs are fast and short acting and as their insulin secretory action is glucose dependent, they are less likely to cause hypoglycemia as compared to SU. Incidence of hypoglycemia is 0.6% for repaglinide and 1% for nateglinide as against 10% with SU.

These agents are relatively safe in patients with renal failure. Incidence of skin rash is very low with these agents. So far there is no head-to-head comparison of glinides and SU as far as weight gain, hypoglycemia and overall efficacy are concerned.

These agents are not recommended for patients below 18 years of age. They have not been tested in pregnant women.

## SUMMARY

- Fast acting and have short duration of action.
- Enhance impaired 1st phase of insulin release.
- Main effect is controlling PP hyperglycemia.

- Less risk of hypoglycemia.
- One tablet per meal offers flexibility in life-style.
- Long-term benefits with these drugs are being investigated.
- These drugs are relatively expensive.
- They have got some role in cases with renal impairment.

# Chapter 11

# Metformin

This drug belongs to Biguanide group of oral hypoglycemic agents. Other molecules from this group—Phenformin and buformin—are no longer available because of their serious side effect, mainly lactic acidosis. Although the molecule was introduced in middle of 20th century, it was used widely only for nearly two decades. Initially, it was not liberally used in western world due to fear of lactic acidosis till the end of 20th century. After the release of UKPDS results this molecule has received good acknowledgment in medical field.

## MECHANISM OF ACTION

Metformin is not clearly understood till today. It acts mainly by improving insulin resistance at hepatic level. It increases glucose utilization mainly through non-oxidative pathways. Other actions of metformin include activation of AMP protein kinase, stimulation tyrosine kinase activity and translocation of GLUT 1.

Metformin monotherapy reduces HbA1C by 1.4 to 2.0% and reduced F BSL by 50-90 mg%. This drug does not induce hyperinsulinemia. In fact in some cases it may result in fall in insulin levels.

## CLINICAL USAGE

It is useful as monotherapy to reduce hyperglycemia in those patients in whom life-style modification has failed to achieve normal glucose level. It is especially useful in overweight cases. It can be administered as immediate release tablet twice or thrice daily or sustained release tablet once daily. With the use of sustained release metformin tablets, the peak plasma level of the drug achieved is 25% higher and the peak is delayed by 4 hours, as compared to immediate release metformin tablet. It is excreted unchanged in urine by tubular excretion.

The tablet should be given with meal and one should start with a smaller dose in order to avoid adverse effects, which include nausea, anorexia, vomiting and diarrhea. Some patients notice the outer shell of the extended release tablet in stools and raise doubts whether the active ingredient of the tablet has been absorbed or not. These patients need proper reassurance.

Incidence of hypoglycemia is about 10% in metformin users.

Risk of lactic acidosis with use of metformin in otherwise healthy diabetics is practically nil as metformin increases lactate oxidation. Overall incidence of lactic acidosis in metformin users is 3 per 100000 patient–years. Mean plasma lactate level was found to be similar in metformin users and non-users. The risk of lactic acidosis in high when metformin is given to patients with renal failure, hepatic failure or heart failure, sepsis, tissue hypoxia, alcoholic person or patient with severe dehydration.

Metformin should be stopped for one day prior to and two days after the radiological procedure involving iodinated dye.

Some patients experience B12 deficiency with chronic metformin use. But routine B12 supplementation with metformin is not justified.

Apart from glucose-lowering effect this drug has got multiple additional beneficial effects in a diabetic person. Use of this drug results in some reduction in weight. Degree of weight loss is up to 3% of baseline weight. The effect is seen within 6 months of drug therapy.

*Mechanisms of weight loss with metformin are*:
- Increased thermogenic activity in brown adipose tissues
- Reduced food intake
- Increase in futile substrate cycling
- Enhanced carbohydrate utilization
- Reduction in hyperinsulinemia.

Metformin reduces serum triglycerides and to some extent lowers total cholesterol and LDL cholesterol. It accelerates fibrinolytic response in diabetic person.

All these effects result in improving cardiovascular outcome in type II diabetes. UKPDS results mention that this is the only hypoglycemic agent, which has shown reduction in macrovascular complications in type II diabetes. It has been suggested that metformin acts by modifying various non-traditional risk factors along with its effect on standard risk factors.

Metformin has some role in children with type II diabetes. It is useful in overweight type I diabetics to reduce their insulin dosage.

## METFORMIN IN COMBINATION

This molecule can be safely combined with other hypoglycemic agents.

It has been successfully combined with controlled particle-size glibenclamide though glitazones and metformin act by reducing insulin resistance; these agents can be combined safely because the sites of action of these agents are different. Glitazones act at skeletal muscles and adipose tissues while metformin acts mainly at liver cells. This drug has been successfully used in combination with recent oral antidiabetic agents like DPP IV inhibitors (Sitagliptin/ Vildagliptin).

In some cases use of triple combination (metformin + glitazone + glibenclamide/glimeperide) are found to be necessary, when adequate glycemic control is not achieved with two agents.

Metformin can be combined with insulin in both type I and type II diabetics to reduce insulin dosage. Interestingly this is achieved without hypoglycemia. Metformin addition helps in reducing weight and cholesterol in these cases.

## OTHER USES

- As primary prevention of type II diabetes in patients with IGT – Diabetes prevention program (DPP).
- In women with polycystic ovarian disease (PCOD). Metformin reduces insulin resistance and induces ovulation and fertility. Dose recommended is 1.5 gm/day for 6 months, followed by Clomiphene for 3 months.
- It has some role in reducing abdominal obesity and correcting lipodystrophy in AIDS cases treated with antiretroviral agents.

## SUMMARY

- Metformin acts by reducing insulin resistance.
- It reduces both micro- and macrovascular complications of diabetes.
- It can be safely combined with other oral agents and with insulin.

- The benefits are additive after combining these agents.
- Availability of extended release form of metformin has reduced side-effects and has improved adherence to treatment.
- It is contraindicated in patients with renal/hepatic/cardiac failure/conditions associated with tissue hypoxia.
- Use of metformin in pregnancy is not recommended.

Chapter 12

# Alpha Glucosidase Inhibitors

Controlling postprandial (PP) hyperglycemia without inducing hypoglycemia is a challenging task is some diabetic patients. PP hyperglycemia is found to be associated with higher cardiovascular morbidity in diabetic population. Hypoglycemic agents like SU or metformin control mainly fasting hyperglycemia with relatively less benefit on PP hyperglycemia. Dietary modification involving higher percentage of fiber and complex carbohydrates is associated with poor adherence.

The need for agents that specifically target PP hyperglycemia is met by short acting insulin analogues, glinides and alpha glucosidase inhibitors (AGI). Three molecules are available from AGI group-acarbose, miglitol, and voglibose.

## DOSAGE OF AGENTS FROM AGI GROUP

- *Acarbose*: The oldest AGI is acarbose. Dose is 25 mg BID to maximum of 100 mg TID.
- *Miglitol*: It came after acarbose. Dose is 25 mg BID to maximum of 100 mg TID.
- *Voglibose*: It is the new entrant in this group. It has got relatively less GI side effect. Dose is 0.2 mg BID to maximum of 0.3 mg TID.

## MECHANISM OF ACTION

These drugs competitively block the intestinal enzyme required for breaking down complex carbohydrates to simple sugars, which are then easily absorbed from intestines. Competitive inhibition of these enzymes leads to slow digestion of carbohydrates, thereby blunting the postprandial excursions of blood glucose. These agents have very high affinity for the enzymes but the process is reversible. These drugs act mainly at intestinal wall and they have hardly any systemic action.

They are poorly absorbed from intestinal tract. They are metabolized in large intestine.

## CLINICAL ASPECTS

Ideally, these agents should be taken at 1st bite of food or within 15 minutes of meal.

They reduce PP blood sugar by approximately 50 mg%. The reduction in HbA1C is about 0.7%. They are weight neutral. Hypoglycemia is uncommon with these agents when used alone.

But when these agents are used with other hypoglycemic agents, especially SU, then hypoglycemia can occur and could be severe. Whenever, a patient is being treated with AGI, he must always carry glucose powder or tablets with his for combating hypoglycemic episode. Sucrose or cane sugar if given to these patients, is not digested speedily enough due to mode of action of these drugs; hence sucrose is of no use for treating acute hypoglycemic spell.

Main side effects are flatulence and bloating. These side effects are socially unacceptable and are the main cause of lack of adherence. Always start with a lower dose. Gradually increasing the dose as per the individual patient tolerance will improve adherence. Elevation of liver enzymes is noted with use of these agents.

AGI can be combined with SU, glitazones, metformin and insulin with significant additive effect. These agents are specifically useful in elderly diabetics, who have associated constipation. They are useful in preventing type II diabetes in patients with IGT.

AGI have some role to play in type I diabetics through their insulin sparing effect. When combined with insulin in type I cases, insulin dose is reduced nearly by 1/3. They provide smother glycemic control and have less incidence of hypoglycemia, when combined with insulin. Additional reduction in HbA1C is about 0.5% when these agents are added to insulin.

## CONTRAINDICATIONS

- Malabsorption syndrome, intestinal obstruction
- Hepatic diseases
- Severe renal impairment
- Pregnancy and lactating mothers
- Age less than 12 years.

## ROLE OF AGI IN THERAPY

As a monotherapy, they are useful in recently detected type II diabetics who have minimally raised blood sugar levels. They are specifically useful in elderly population. At times they are of use when other OHA produce significant side effects or are contraindicated.

They can be nicely combined with other OHA and with insulin.

Chapter 13

# Thiazolidinediones—Insulin Sensitizers

*Unique group of drugs*—Thiazolidinediones/glitazones/TZD—that is available for nearly a decade has given a new direction to diabetes care. These drugs modify one of the basic pathophysiological feature of type II diabetes, i.e. insulin resistance. These drugs when used alone or in combination reduce blood sugar and improve glycemic control. Two molecules are available—Pioglitazone and Rosiglitazone. The original glitazone—Troglitazone has been withdrawn from market due to its idiosyncratic severe hepatic damage.

These drugs act by stimulating nuclear receptor PPAR $\gamma$, which results in complex intracellular mechanism involving expression of various genes, ultimately resulting in reduction of insulin resistance at skeletal muscles, liver and adipose tissues. By reducing insulin resistance they improve peripheral glucose uptake in both lean and obese insulin resistant type II diabetics by nearly 30-100%. Use of these drugs results in reduction in free fatty acids too. These drugs raise adiponectin levels.

They increase beta cell function by nearly 50%. They produce higher insulin response in presence of relatively lower blood glucose concentration. This effect is due to fall in glucose toxicity and improvement in insulin sensitivity.

## CLINICAL USE OF TZD

Rosiglitazone and pioglitazone are widely used in management of type II diabetes. These agents reduce insulin resistance; improve peripheral glucose utilization in both lean and obese insulin resistant type II diabetics by nearly 30-100%.

They reduce F BSL by nearly 60 mg% and reduce A1C by 1.4%. Usual starting dose of rosiglitazone is 2 mg twice daily, maximum dose is 8 mg per day. Staring dose of pioglitazone is 15 mg and maximum dose is 45 mg per day. Dosage increment should be carried out only after 2 weeks interval.

These agents can be combined with sulfonylureas, metformin, DPP IV inhibitors and insulin. Combination with metformin is especially in obese patients. These agents are routinely used in various triple drug combinations available in India.

Pioglitazone improves lipid profile- reduces triglycerides by 9%, raises HDL by 12-19% and reduce density of LDL. Rosiglitazone raise LDL levels. Use of rosiglitazone and CV mortality is heavily debated topic in the world. Many Indian patients have raised triglycerides and low HDL. This typical Indian-dyslipidemic pattern is aggravated by rosiglitazone—a clinical observation noted in our day-to-day practice. Effects of Glitazones on lipoprotein (a)-(Lp-a) is variable in different studies.

These agents help in redistribution of adipose tissues. They reduce visceral adiposity and increase subcutaneous fat. They improve insulin sensitivity of hepatic cells and peripheral tissues

Microalbuminuria, urinary albumin excretion and urinary endothelin are reduced after regular use of TZD. Modest reduction in Blood Pressure (6-8 mm of Hg) is seen after use of these drugs.

These drugs have got favorable effects on endothelium, VSMC, platelets and macrophage, thereby improving stability of atherosclerotic plaque. Reduction in carotid intima-medial thickness is seen in some studies after use of these agents.

All the benefits mentioned above work together to improve CV morbidity in diabetes. Incidence of coronary re-stenosis is found to lower in patients on TZD.

## SIDE EFFECTS OF TZD

- If baseline S ALT (S GPT) level is above 2.5 times normal then these agents are contraindicated S ALT. Enzyme levels are monitored once in 2 months for 1st year of therapy and less frequently later on. When the S ALT level goes beyond 3 times normal, these agents are discontinued. At times poorly controlled diabetic person may have moderately elevated S. ALT, which improves with after glycemic control by using glitazones.
- Fluid retention is another important side effect of TZD. This can lead to weight gain of nearly 3 kg. In some cases the weight gain can be up to 8 kg. Fluid retention leads to dilutional anemia, which is normocytic and normochromic.
- Glitazones are not to be used in cases with NYHA class III and IV cardiac failure cases. These agents are to be given with caution in patients with class II and class I cardiac failure. Staring dose should be lower than usual and up-titration should be gradual.
- These agents modify insulin resistance in patients with PCOD. They can induce ovulation and pregnancy. Women during child- bearing period who are given these drugs should be asked to use contraceptive methods (preferably physical barrier) concomitantly in order to

avoid unplanned pregnancy and effects of medication on fetus.

### Drug Interactions

Pioglitazone is metabolized by cytochrome P450 isoform CYP3A4 and rosiglitazone is metabolized by CYP2C8 isoform. Pioglitazone has got important drug interactions with alprazolam, carbamazepine, cisapride, diltiazem, diazepam, cyclosporin, fexofenadine, felodipine, midazolam, nifedipine, quinine, simvastatin, tacrolimus and verapamil as these drugs are metabolized by CYP3A4 isoform. Ketoconazole inhibits activity of CYP3A4 isoform and concomitant use of pioglitazone with this drug raises the possibility of hepatic damage.

Pioglitazone reduce concentration of oral contraceptives (OC) by nearly 30%, thereby reducing efficacy of these agents. In such cases OC with higher hormonal concentration or other methods of contraception should be recommended.

As opposed to pioglitazone, rosiglitazone is found to have no major drug interactions with commonly used drugs.

Large dosage of aspirin increase insulin secretion by inhibition of prostaglandin E2. Co-administration of glitazones can result in hypoglycemia.

## SUMMARY

These drugs reduce insulin resistance, and provide multiple benefits like glucose control, improving lipid profile, lowering of blood pressure, and improving endothelial function. All of them help in cardiovascular outcome in a diabetic patient.

Some weight gain and edema is expected with these agents.

Hypoglycemia is less frequent with TZD when used alone.

Liver enzymes should be monitored when these agents are prescribed.

Watch carefully for signs and symptoms of CCF when the patient is on TZD.

# Chapter 14

# Incretin-based Therapies

Although SU and metformin are widely used drugs in diabetes, they have their own limitations like risk of hypoglycemia, weight gain, controlling mainly fasting hyperglycemia and GI intolerance. The need for a new drug, which will take care of these shortcomings of existing agents, is partly met by new class of agents called incretin agonists.

(Exenatide and Liraglutide) and incretin enhancers (Sitagliptin and Vildagliptin).

## INCRETIN EFFECT

This effect was described nearly 3 decades ago. It was noted that blood glucose control after oral glucose intake was mainly because of increased insulin secretion that was not observed with intravenous glucose infusion. The difference in amount of insulin secretion after oral and intravenous glucose administration in iso-glycemic studies is called as incretin effect. This effect is mediated by 2 important gut-hormones namely GLP-1 (Glucagon Like Peptide-1) and GIP (Glucose Dependent Insulinotropic Polypeptide)

*Major effects of these hormones are*:

- Stimulation of insulin secretion in glucose dependent manner.
- Inhibition of gastric emptying, I.
- Inducing early satiety.
- Promote weight loss in diabetic patients.
- Suppression of glucagon secretion after meals.

In patients with IGT or type II diabetes, GLP-1 levels are reduced by 20-30%. GIP levels are not reduced in these patients but action of GIP is reduced (GIP resistance).

GLP-1 is rapidly degraded by an enzyme called dipeptidyl peptidase-4 (DPP-IV). This limits the duration of action of GLP-1 to 2-3 minutes. DPP is a protease protein-digesting enzyme, present both in circulation and on cell membrane.

Incretin based therapies are subdivided into two groups:

- GLP-1 agonists (Exenatide)
- Incretin enhancers (DPP-IV inhibitors).

## GLP-1 AGONISTS (EXENATIDE)

GLP-1 agonist available today is exenatide (Byetta or Increnat) is synthetic exendin-4, exendin-4 is found in saliva of a lizard -Gila monster. Amino acid sequence of exendin-4 is similar to that of human GLP-1. It binds to GLP-1 receptor and does have almost all actions of GLP-1.

Exenatide has to be administered by subcutaneous injection. It's peak action and half-life is 2 hours. Main action of drug is seen up to 6 hours and no drug is detected after 10 hours of injection. In type II diabetes, Exenatide completely reverses defect in 1st phase of insulin secretion, and augments second phase of insulin secretion too.

Exenatide has short duration of action. Hence, the main benefit is control of post-prandial hyperglycemia. As its action diminishes after 8-10 hours, it has got no effect on fasting hyperglycemia. It is to be given 30 –60 minutes before meal. It has to be given twice daily. Usual dose is 5 –10 mcg.

Exenatide is approved for use in combination with SU and metofrmin. Reduction in HbA1C with this combination is about 1% and there is significant weight loss.

Apart from reduction in blood glucose, Exenatide has got favorable effect on traditional cardiovascular risk factors like lipid profile, blood pressure, CRP and ALT.

Major side effect of exenatide is nausea that is seen in 50% of patients. About 5% of cases stop exenatide because of nausea. Starting dose of 5 mcg helps in reducing nausea. It can be gradually stepped up to 10 mcg.

Other side effects are hypoglycemia (especially when used with SU), pancreatitis, development of antibodies to exenatide, (significance not clearly known).

Long acting incretin agonist is just round the corner. It can be administered once a week. Incidence of nausea is less with this drug.

## INCRETIN ENHANCERS (DPP-IV INHIBITORS)

Sitagliptin and vildagliptin are available DPP-IV inhibitors today. Alogliptin and saxagliptin are yet to come. These molecules inhibit action DPP-IV thereby elevate GLP-1 and GIP. Inhibition is prolonged 12-24 hours. These agents reduce both fasting and PP hyperglycemia. Reduction in HbA1C is about 0.7%. Usual dose of sitagliptin is 100 mg once daily and that of vildagliptin is 50 mg twice daily. Incase of renal impairment the dose of Sitagliptin is reduced.

These drugs can be safely combined with metformin. The reduction in HbA1C is about 2% with this combination. Vildagliptin has been successfully combined with SU, AGI, glitazones and insulin with additive benefits. In type I diabetics vildagliptin can be combined with insulin. It results in better glycemic control with reduction of insulin dose and with less incidence of hypoglycemia.

Adverse effects of these drugs are recurrent nasopharyngitis or urinary infection and headache. Hypoglycemia is common when vildagliptin is used with SU.

In animal studies these agents have shown increase in beta cell mass, increase in beta cell proliferation and reduction in beta cell apoptosis. It is hoped that these actions will be demonstrated in humans too. It might modify the progression of type II diabetes.

As on today these drugs are costly. Hence they are not used liberally in all diabetics. These drugs have potential benefit for rejuvenating dying beta cells. Future studies will demonstrate whether these agents are of any use in providing "cure" for diabetes—a dream that every diabetic person has in his mind.

Chapter 15

# Insulin Use in Diabetics

More than 75 years have passed since this highly effective drug-insulin for control of hyperglycemia was invented. Major advances in insulin were for last 2-3 decades. Initially available impure insulin from animal origin has now been replaced by genetically engineered r-DNA insulin, which is pure and less immunogenic.

Insulin is a must for all type I diabetics and many type II diabetics who do not achieve adequate glucose control with oral hypoglycemic agents. Insulin is recommended during management of GDM. Stressful period in a type II diabetic person like acute infection, myocardial infarction, trauma, surgical procedure, cerebrovascular accident will demand insulin for tight control of blood glucose level. Patients with renal failure or hepatic failure are often managed beautifully with insulin especially with analogues.

Indications of insulin

| | |
|---|---|
| Long-term | • Type I diabetes<br>• Type II diabetes having poor control with OHA<br>• Chronic renal/ Hepatic failure |
| Short-term | • GDM<br>• Infections<br>• Myocardial infarction<br>• Cerebrovascular accident<br>• Perioperative period<br>• Trauma<br>• Acute renal or hepatic failure |

## TYPES OF INSULIN

### Based on Pharmacokinetics

Rapid acting, short acting, intermediate acting and long acting.

Action profile of various insulin preparations

| *Insulin preparation* | *Onset of action* | *Peak of action* | *Duration of action* |
|---|---|---|---|
| Rapid acting insulin | | | |
| Lispro | 5-15 min | 30-90 min | 3-5 hrs |
| Novorapid | 5-15 min | 30-90 min | 3-5 hrs |
| Apidra | 5-15 min | 30-90 min | 3-5 hrs |
| Short acting | | | |
| Regular | 30-60 min | 2-3 hrs | 5-8 hrs |
| Intermediate acting | | | |
| NPH | 2-4 hrs | 4-10 hrs | 10-16 hrs |
| Lente | 3-4 hrs | 4-12 hrs | 12-18 hrs |
| Long acting | | | |
| Ultralente | 6-10 hrs | 10-16 hrs | 18-24 hrs |
| Glargine | 2-4 hrs | No peak | 20-24 hrs |
| Detemir | 2-4 hrs | 6-14 hrs | 16-20 hrs |
| Insulin mixtures | | | |
| 30/70 human mix 30% regular, 70% NPH | 30-60 min | Double peak | 10-16 hrs |
| 50/50 human mix 50% of Regular & NPH | 30-60 min | Double peak | 10-16 hrs |
| 50/50 Lispro mix 50% of lispro and Intermediate | 5-15 min | Double peak | 12-20 hrs |
| 25/75 Lispro mix 25% lispro, 75% Intermediate | 5-15 min | Double peak | 12-20 hrs |
| 30/70 Novomix 30% Novorapid, 70% Intermediate | 5-15 min | Double peak | 12-20 hrs |

### Based on Concentration–40 U/ml,100 U/ml, 500 U/ml

Many of our patients are familiar with U40 insulin vials and U40 insulin syringes. At times they get U100 syringes from a relative or a friend staying abroad. If they continue to use U40 insulin with U100 syringe, they lose glucose control, as they are under-insulinized. On the contrary if somebody is prescribed U100 insulin (to meet very high insulin need or to save cost) and he continues to use U40 syringe then he is bound to get hypoglycemia. Insulin concentration and the syringe strength must match with each other—like sari and a blouse. Mix and match policy does not work well here.

There are many reasons why syringes are the most common way to take insulin:

- Syringes are the least expensive form of insulin delivery available.
- Syringes are reliable, with very simple moving parts
- Syringes come in several sizes, with a variety of needle lengths and gauges (thickness).
- Syringes are easy to use and learning how to use them is simple.
- Syringes are stocked by almost every pharmacy or drug store.
- Syringes give you access to all insulin types.
- If you need to inject two types of insulin that can be combined, syringes allow you to combine them in one injection.
- Syringes are generally covered by insurance plans that cover prescription products.

One should be extra careful about confirming the fact that the patient is using proper syringe for the insulin he has been prescribed.

### Compare and Contrast

As all the insulin brands available today are using r-DNA technology and are providing 'HUMAN' insulin and these preparations are in very pure form, the discussion on species of insulin and purity of insulin has now become obsolete.

Insulin can be given to the patient either to supplement basal insulin secretion or to supplement prandial insulin secretion or to both. Patients with type I diabetes need both basal and prandial insulin. Type II diabetics need only basal

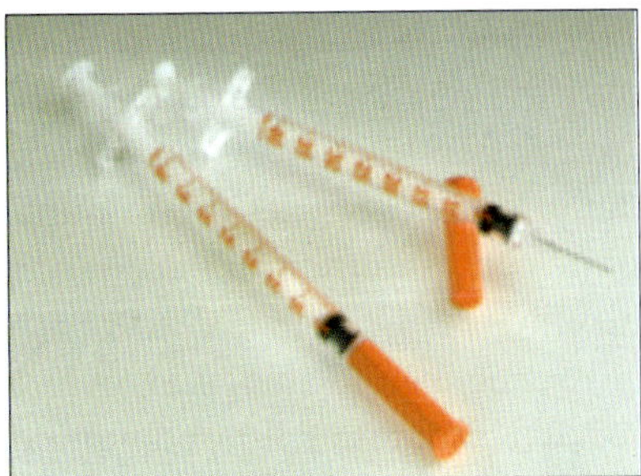

**Figure 15.1:** U40 syringe with red cap

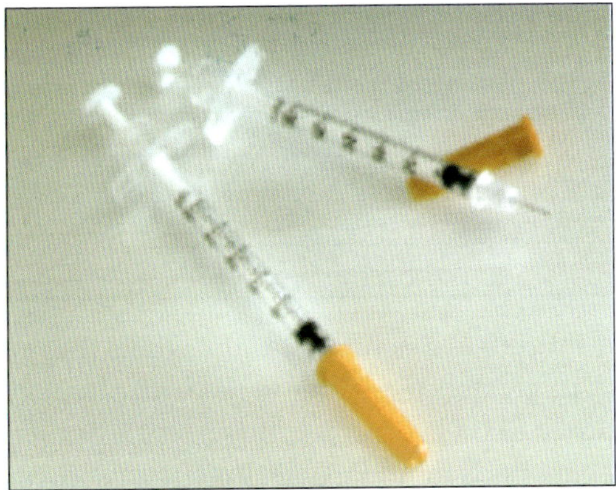

**Figure 15.2:** U100 syringe with orange cap

insulin supplement for few years, but later on they too need prandial insulin dosage.

Basal insulin therapy can be administered by giving one or rarely two injections of long acting insulin. Peakless insulin is preferred over NPH as it provides optimal basal insulin supplementation with minimal risk of hypoglycemia. If the insulin need is high then it is advised to split the dose into two halves-50% at breakfast, 50% after dinner.

NPH can be used as basal insulin if there are cost constraints. But the results achieved with NPH are sub-optimal and the risk of hypoglycemia is high. It has to be given twice daily. Some countries use multiple small doses of NPH to mimic continuous basal insulin secretion.

Prandial insulin supplementation can be best achieved by giving rapid acting insulin analogues before meals. Dose of insulin is decided by amount of carbohydrates in the meal. Less optimal results can be achieved by short acting regular insulin given 20-30 minutes prior to meal. But this can result in more number of hypoglycemic episodes.

Insulin use in type I diabetics is aimed at achieving target blood as below

| | |
|---|---|
| Preprandial | 70-130 mg% |
| 1 hour postprandial | 100-180 mg% |
| 2 hour postprandial | 80-150 mg% |
| 3 AM | 100-140 mg% |

These targets are achieved only when the patient is educated, motivated and is able to recognize hypoglycemia. He should do SMBG very often. Suggested insulin program for these patients is multiple daily doses of insulin injections (MDII) with basal insulin. Usual starting dose is 0.5 to 1.0 U per kg bodyweight. The dose is increased during intercurrent illness and prepubertal growth spurt. Dose is reduced during honeymoon phase of type I diabetics.

Half of the total daily dose is given as basal insulin and remaining half is distributed amongst multiple doses of rapid acting insulin analogues depending upon amount of carbohydrates in each meal (1-1.5 U per 10 gm of carbohydrate). Dose of basal insulin dose is adjusted by monitoring fasting blood sugar after 3-4 days. Dose of preprandial insulin is adjusted as per blood sugar levels. Prebreakfast, prelunch and predinner dose of rapid acting analogue insulin is lowered or stepped up if prelunch, predinner or bedtime blood sugars are low or high, as compared to recommended targets.

Not all type I diabetics are motivated and carry out SMBG. Less optimal insulin program of insulin can be used for them. It includes:

- Two injections per day–Split mix regimen, Short acting and intermediate acting insulin, mixed and given before breakfast and before dinner.
- Three injections per day–Mixed insulin at breakfast, then short acting before dinner and intermediate insulin at bedtime.

The situation is slightly simpler in type II diabetics. They have blunted or absent 1st phase insulin response to meal, insulin resistance and beta cell dysfunction leading to limited insulin secretory capacity. Fortunately insulin resistance and beta cell dysfunction improves after controlling hyperglycemia with exogenous insulin.

Targets of blood sugar in type II diabetics are

| | |
|---|---|
| Fasting | 70 to 100 mg% |
| 2 hour Postprandial | 100 to 180 mg% |
| Bedtime | 100-140 mg% |

Insulin therapy is modified as per blood sugar levels. Basal insulin along-with OHA is enough for those who have fasting BSL in between 110 – 180 mg%. Usual starting dose of glargine is 10 U at bedtime. In patients in whom fasting blood sugar is above 180 mg% insulin requirement is high (1.5 U/kg) during initial phase of therapy. Both basal and prandial insulin are needed to achieve normoglycemia. Later on dose of insulin can be reduced to 1 U/kg/day. In those with very severe diabetes (fasting BSL above 300 mg% or those who have profound insulin deficiency, are managed as type I diabetics. They need MDI and basal insulin with frequent blood sugar monitoring.

It must be informed clearly to the patient that insulin therapy must be accompanied by strict diet, regular physical activity and total abstinence from tobacco, in order to obtain desired benefits.

Gradually insulin therapy corrects underlying defects in type II diabetes and then these patients can be shifted back to oral agents with life style modification. Patient should be told that if insulin is started during early phase of disease then it might be stopped early. If it is started late in type II diabetes then usually it is continued forever. Therefore every type II diabetic should learn basic aspects of insulin therapy and pick up practical steps about insulin administration, insulin storage, etc.

Use of insulin as a first line therapy in type II diabetics may induce long lasting remission. But this idea is not well appreciated by majority of our patients due to myths and misconceptions about insulin.

Journal of Association of Physicians of India (JAPI) has recommended following guidelines for insulin therapy in Indian patients. In JAPI special issue 2009 February.

- Start with once a day insulin – Premix 30/70, Dose - 10U To be given before breakfast if Predinner blood glucose is high to be given in evening if pre-breakfast blood glucose is high.

- Titrate as per blood glucose level

| *Pre-meal blood glucose in mg/dl* | *Change in insulin dose in units* |
|---|---|
| < 100 | - 2 |
| 100-110 | Nil |
| 110-140 | + 2 |
| 141-180 | + 4 |
| Above 180 | + 6 |

Split the dose in two equal haves, one before breakfast and one before dinner when total daily insulin need goes up beyond 30U.

# Chapter 16

# Insulin Pump Therapy

Diabetes Control and Complications Trial (DCCT) has established the fact that tight glucose control reduces microvascular complications in type I diabetics. Recently, published EDIC trial has shown that glucose memory effect lasts for years together in future, reducing long-term complications. Insulin is normally administered as Multiple Daily Injections (MDI) (Basal-Bolus program), which include 3-4 injections per day.

Another method of providing insulin is Continuous Subcutaneous Insulin Infusion (CSII), which offers more flexible lifestyle to type I diabetic patients as regards their meal timing and meal composition. Additional 0.5% reduction in A1C is achieved with this mode of insulin delivery. Decrease in insulin requirement is noted in patients using CSII. Overall control is better and chances of severe hypoglycemia are less with CSII.

Insulin delivery is pre-programmed by CSII or pump. It involves two components. First is basal insulin and second is bolus or prandial insulin.

Basal insulin is administered as hourly component. The rate of basal insulin can be altered or can be suspended as per the clinical need. Bolus insulin is pre-programmed as per the carbohydrate ratio and correction factors. Patient has to monitor pre-meal blood sugar. The pump then determines the bolus dose of insulin. Pump has got other features like insulin-on-board, bolus history, mealtime alarm ... all of these reduce the risk of glucose variability. The amount of insulin is less with pump therapy and therefore, it causes less weight gain as opposed to MDI.

Increment in insulin is in smaller proportion as opposed to that in MDI. It helps in reducing risk of severe hypoglycemia. Pump therapy mimics natural insulin secretion and therefore is more accurate. Acceptance of insulin pump is gradually increasing in western world. Situation in India is different because of cost and inadequate motivation.

## INDICATIONS

- Wide fluctuations in blood glucose with MDI.
- Target A1C not achieved with MDI.
- Recurrent hypoglycemia.
- Patient asks for a flexible lifestyle.
- Patients with eating disorders.
- Competitive athletes.
- Infants and neonates.
- Pronounced Dawn's phenomenon.
- Preconception in pregnant adolescent.

## PATIENT SELECTION

Insulin pump therapy is to be given in properly selected patients in order to achieve perfect goal of glucose control. Patient and his family members must be highly motivated to perform at least four blood sugar tests everyday, to record those results in proper format, to have regular follow-up with the health care team. They must have good understanding about diabetes. The initial HbA1C should be preferably below 8.5% but at times those patients who are uncontrolled with MDI can be given a choice of insulin pump therapy. The patient selected should be committed to achieve A1C below 7%.

## TYPES OF INSULIN PUMP

Five major types of insulin pumps are available in market today. They have minor variation in insulin reservoir capacity (180 to 315 units), minimal basal rate increment (0.025 to 1.0 micro units per hour) and minimal bolus dose increment (0.05 to 1.0 micro units per hour). Some features are unique to some brands, e.g. animas ping has got largest display, omnipod offers freestyle glucometer in PDA, disetronic spirit has got customizable menu option, Deltec Cozmo has got facility to provide variable basal rate for each day of the week and meditronic paradigm has got real time CGMS along with the pump.

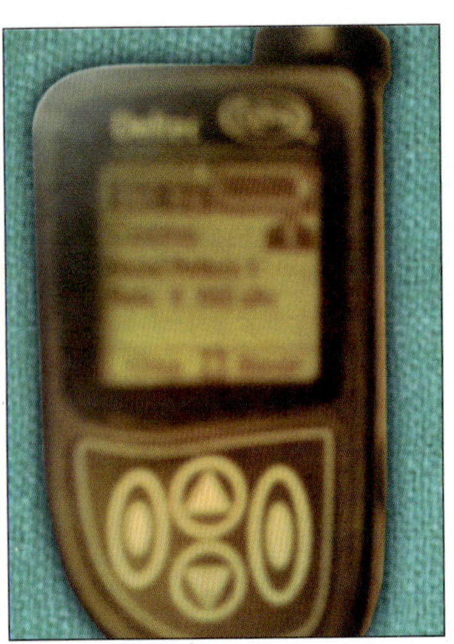

**Figure 16.1:** Deltec Cosmo pump

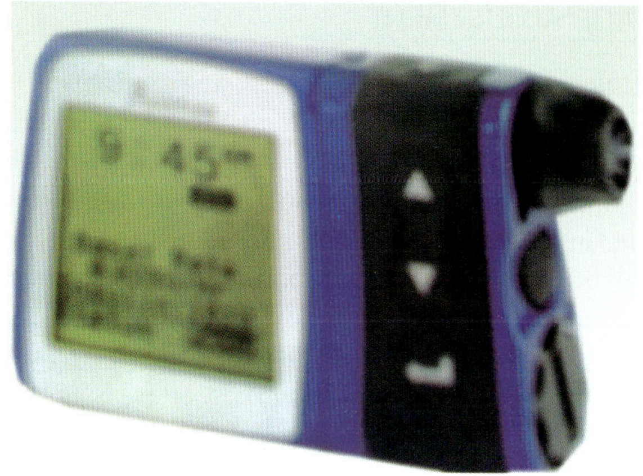

Figure 16.2: Animas pump

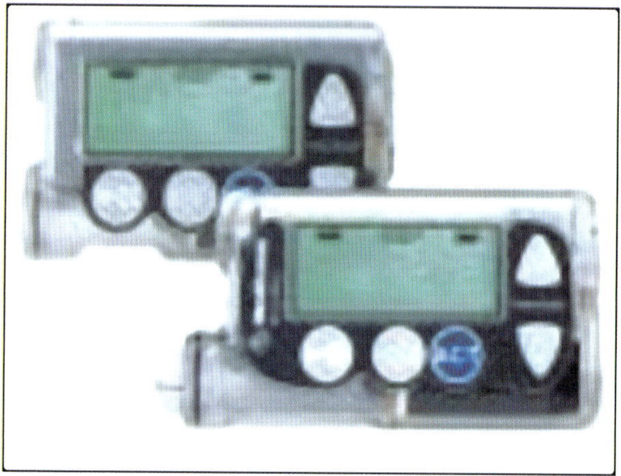

Figure 16.3: Meditronic minimed

## DOSAGE ADJUSTMENT

Initial dose of insulin is usually 0.5 U per kg. Usually when the patient is shifted from MDI to CSII, total daily dose is reduced by 10 to 20%. Half of the total dose is given as bolus and half is given as bolus insulin. Basal dose is further divided into units per hour. Bolus dose consists of meal bolus and a correction bolus. Correction bolus is determined by carbohydrate ratio (500 divided by total daily dose –TDD of insulin) and correction factor (1800 divided by TDD).

Fo rxample, if TDD is 60 U, then basal dose is 30 U, bolus dose is 30 U.

- Basal dose 30 U divided by 24 = 1.2 U per hour
- Bolus dose = Scheduled meal dose + Correction dose

Depending upon blood glucose levels, dose of basal or bolus insulin is adjusted. Former are adjusted as per fasting and nocturnal blood glucose levels. Bolus dose is adjusted as per premeal blood glucose levels.

After the initial setting is done then the patient is normally asked to come for follow-up after 2-3 weeks. Review of his blood glucose profiles, diet adherence is carried out. Signs of local inflammation or hypertrophy at the site of the pump should be examined. Local antibiotic like mupirocin can be applied.

## PROBLEMS WITH PUMP THERAPY

The biggest risk for those on CSII is DKA due to pump failure. The reasons for pump failure include blockage or leakage of tubing, luerlock problems, dislodgement of soft cannula below the skin or entrapment of air in the insulin

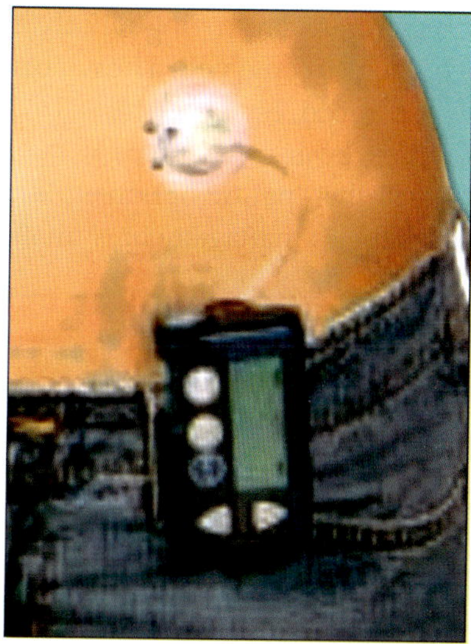

**Figure 16.4:** Pump in use

tubing. At times hypoglycemia can occur but the incidence is low and severity is less as opposed to that with MDI. Patients can have pump-holidays for 2 hours. If the period extends beyond 2 hours then additional dose of insulin is to be given.

Artificial pancreas is a step ahead in diabetes management in which CSII is combined with CGMS (Continuous Glucose Monitoring System). CGMS gives information about rate and direction of glucose levels. Changes in insulin dose and diet can be done accordingly. CGMS usage has produced 0.5% additional reduction in A1C. REAL time CGMS is more accurate and easy to use. Two other models available are Dexcom seven and Abbot Freestyle Navigator.

Diabetes care has been improving rapidly in last decade. Innovative technologies come with a heavy price tag, which not all patients can afford, especially those from developing countries and those who are uninsured. Moreover even after using these hi-tech therapeutic options, place of life-style modification in diabetes management is unaltered.

Chapter 17

# Combined ADA and EASD 2009 Algorithm for Management of Type II Diabetes

## TREATMENT RECOMMENDATIONS FROM ADA/EASD

The updated guidelines from the ADA/EASD recommend that basal insulin and sulfonylureas are specifically recommended as top-tier choices for treating patients, who fail to control their blood sugar with metformin and lifestyle modifications. Another medication should be added to improve glucose control so as to reach an A1c level of below 7.0%.

## BASAL INSULIN

Insulin is the oldest and most effective therapies available for management of hyperglycemia. With aggressive titration, insulin elicits the greatest reduction in A1c levels (typically 1.5 to 3.5%), allowing the majority of patients to reach A1c targets. Formulations of insulin vary in their rate of onset and duration of benefit, with combinations of formulations being appropriate for some patients. However, once-daily basal insulin is generally the starter insulin of choice. One of the beneficial side effects of insulin is the salutary effect that it has on the patient's lipid profile. HDL levels generally increase with treatment, whereas TG levels decline.

But insulin usage is also associated with unwanted side effects, such as weight gain; patients treated with insulin usually gain 2-4 kg for every 1% reduction in A1c. Of additional concern, hypoglycemic events are most common in insulin-treated patients with type I diabetes, but are also a concern for patients with T2DM. A clinical study has shown that the rate of hypoglycemia in those with T2DM is about 30% in those treated with insulin. Severe hypoglycemia, requiring assistance from another person to recognize or treat hypoglycemia, occurred at a rate of 0.5%. Severe hypoglycemia occurred 1-3 times per 100 patient-years of treatment in the insulin treatment group of the UK Prospective Diabetes Study (UKPDS). The incidence of hypoglycemic events varies among the different formulations of insulin. Insulin formulations that are very fast acting and those that are peak-less and long acting are typically linked with the lowest risk for hypoglycemia.

Sulfonylureas are the other class of agents recommended in tier 1 when lifestyle modification and metformin fail to achieve glycemic goals. Sulfonylureas lower blood sugar levels by enhancing the secretion of insulin from the beta cells of the pancreas. Like metformin, sulfonylureas can reduce A1c levels by about 1.5%. The most common side effects accompanying sulfonylurea therapy are hypoglycemia and modest weight gain. Hypoglycemia is more common with the longer-acting sulfonylureas, such as chlorpropamide and glyburide (glibenclamide), than it is with gliclazide, glimepiride, and glipizide. On the basis of this observation, the ADA/EASD recommends against using glyburide (glibenclamide) or chlorpropamide.

The weight gain that is associated with sulfonylurea therapy is generally less than that seen with insulin. Patients treated with sulfonylureas typically gain an average of about 2 kg. Also, the glucose-lowering effects of sulfonylureas appear to be less durable than that of insulin sensitizers.

One study raised the concern that sulfonylureas may increase cardiovascular risks, but that observation has not been supported by the data from other large studies.

Although insulin and sulfonylureas are the most highly recommended choices for patients who fail to achieve A1c targets, the revised ADA/EASD guidelines offer additional recommendations. One of these options is the GLP-1 receptor agonist-exenatide. It is not linked to hypoglycemia, unless used with sulfonylurea. Treatment with the TZD pioglitazone is associated with reduced risk for myocardial infarction as well as improvement in blood lipid profiles. The new revision of the ADA/EASD treatment recommendations offers additional support for considering exenatide and pioglitazone to manage diabetes.

ADA/EASD has recommended GLP-1 receptor agonists as an appropriate alternative for patients in whom avoidance of hypoglycemia and weight gain is desirable. The GLP-1 receptor agonist exenatide offers specific benefits to many patients with T2DM. Unlike basal insulin, sulfonylureas, and TZD, which can all lead to weight gain, treatment with exenatide is associated with weight loss. With

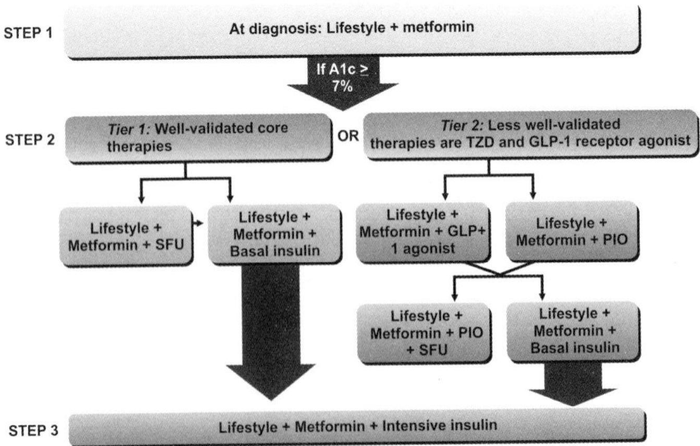

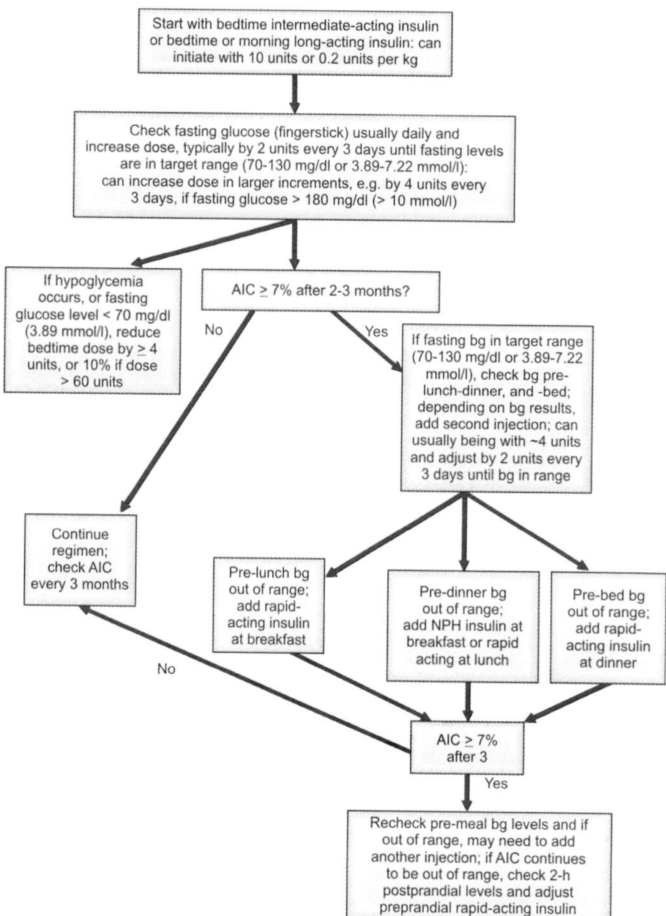


the consequences of obesity and overweight in the diabetic population, exenatide offers an important treatment alternative.

Summary of glucose-lowering interventions

| *Intervention* | *Expected decrease in A1C with monotherapy (%)* | *Advantages* | *Disadvantages* |
|---|---|---|---|
| | | **Tier 1: Well-validated core** | |
| | | **Step 1: Initial therapy** | |
| Lifestyle to decrease weight and increase activity | 1.0-2.0 | Broad benefits | Insufficient for most within first year |
| Metformin | 1.0-2.0 | Weight neutral contraindicated with | GI side effects, renal insufficiency |
| | | **Step 2: Additional therapy** | |
| Insulin | 1.5-3.5 | No dose limit, rapidly effective, improved lipid profile | 1-4 injections daily, monitoring, weight gain, hypoglycemia, analogues are costlier. |
| Sulfonylurea | 1.0-2.0 | Rapidly effective | Weight gain, hypoglycemia (especially with glibenclamide or chlorpropamide) |
| | | **Tier 2: Less well validated** | |
| TZD | 0.5-1.4 | Improved lipid profile (Pioglitazone), potential decrease in MI (Pioglitazone) | Fluid retention, CHF, weight gain, bone fractures, expensive, potential increase in MI (Rosiglitazone) |
| GLP-1 receptor agonist | 0.5-1.0 | Weight loss | Two injections daily, frequent GI side effects, long-term safety not established, expensive |
| | | **Other therapies** | |
| Alpha-glucosidase inhibitor | 0.5-0.8 | Weight neutral | Frequent GI side effects, 3 times/day dosing, expensive |
| Glinide | 0.5-1.5 | Rapidly effective | Weight gain, 3 times/day dosing, hypoglycemia, expensive |
| Pramlintide | 0.5-1.0 | Weight loss | Three injections daily, frequent GI side effects, long-term safety not established, expensive |
| DPP-4 inhibitor | 0.5-0.8 | Weight neutral | Long-term safety not established, expensive |

Chapter 18

# Hypertension and Diabetes

Nearly 50 percent of diabetics are known to have hypertension. The reasons could be:

- Feature of metabolic syndrome and insulin resistance
- Renal dysfunction due to diabetes
- Other causes of hypertension, e.g. renal artery stenosis, Primary hyperaldoseronism, Cushing's syndrome, etc.

## CLINICAL ASPECTS

The target goal for blood pressure in a diabetic person is 130/80. If there is albuminuria, then the goal changes to 125/75 mm of Hg. Target for older people is 150/80 mm Hg.

Blood pressure should be recorded in sitting, supine and in standing position in order to detect postural hypotension—a feature of autonomic neuropathy. Proper cuff size and position of applying the cuff should be ensured. The position of manometer should be at the level of the heart and the patient's arm should be in a relaxed position.

Office blood pressure recording should be accompanied by readings of home blood pressure monitoring by using mercury manometer and stethoscope. This gives important information to clinician about readings at various periods of day/night, thereby guiding him about proper timing of hypotensive medications. Electronic Blood pressure apparatuses available in market are expensive and need frequent calibration.

Ambulatory blood pressure monitoring can be used to find out diurnal variation in blood pressure, especially during sleep. Some diabetics do not show night-time drop in blood pressure. These are called non-dippers and they carry higher mortality as compared to dippers. Ambulatory BP monitoring is useful to diagnose or rule out white-coat hypertension. Blood pressure taken correctly by a primary care physician is also of great value to detect white-coat hypertension.

## MANAGEMENT OF HYPERTENSION

Includes life style modification and medications.

### Lifestyle Changes

Life style changes are aimed at modest weight reduction and controlling adiposity.

*Dietary changes*: Around 500 calories are cut down from the baseline diet of the patient. Food items with low Glycemic Index are preferred. Protein content of diet can be raised to 30% of total calories.

Low salt diet is recommended. Cooking salt is allowed but no added salt is permitted. Items which contain high amount of salt like Pickles, Pappad, potato chips (Wafers), Salted biscuits and canned or packed foods with sodium mono-glutamate, foods with aginomoto should be avoided as far as possible. Black salt (*Saindhav)* can be used in place of salt. Low salt diet restores nocturnal dipping in salt sensitive patients.

Trans-fats are totally banned in hypertensive diabetics and saturated fats should not exceed 7-10% of total fats. PUFA and MUFA fats are preferable. Fried food should be avoided as far as possible. Use of select fruits and majority of vegetables should be encouraged in these patients.

Daily exercise for 60 minutes consisting of stretching, aerobics and resistance training is highly recommended. One should go slow and steady while doing these exercises.

Tobacco use in any form is not allowed. If a person is used to take alcohol then it should be restricted to 2 drinks per day for men and 1 drink/day for women. As alcohol consumption leads to rise in blood pressure and dyslipidemia, one should never suggest use of alcohol (in any form) as a cardio protective agent.

#### Medications for Hypertension

As blood pressure is dependent upon cardiac output (Heart rate X Stroke volume) and peripheral vascular resistance, drugs that modify any of the above parameter will induce change in blood pressure.

Beta-blockers reduce heart rate while diuretics; Natriuretics and Aldosterone antagonists reduce stroke volume. Total peripheral resistance is reduced by calcium channel blockers (CCB), angiotensin converting enzyme inhibitors (ACE inhibitors), angiotensin receptor blockers (ARBs), centrally acting drugs, alpha blockers and nitric oxide enhancers.

All diabetics with proteinuria should be on ACE inhibitors (Ramipril, Lisinopril). Major side effects of these drugs are dry cough, 1st dose hypotension, hyperkalemia and rise in creatinine. Electrolytes and creatinine should be measured 2 weeks and frequently later on, after putting the patient on these drugs.

ARBs (Telmisartan, Losartan, Olmesartan) are useful alternative to ACE inhibitors. As per results of on-target study, combined use of these agents yield slightly inferior results.

Amlodipine or S-Amlodipine can be used when proteiuria/blood pressure remain uncontrolled with maximum dose of ACE Inhibitors or ARB. They are useful in patients having peripheral vascular disease.

Person having IHD should be given beta-blockers. carvedilol, nebivolol and metoprolol are preferred agents.

Patients with congestive heart failure should be given diuretics, carvedilol or aldosterone—antagonists.

Over a period of time one single agent is insufficient to control blood pressure and gradually most of the diabetics need 3-4 hypotensive drugs to achieve the target BP.

Ideally, most of the hypotensive drugs (except diuretics) should be given at night-time in order to correct non-dipping and to prevent early morning rise in BP.

## SUMMARY

- Target BP in diabetics is 130 /80 mm Hg.
- Home monitoring should be encouraged using mercury manometer.
- Ambulatory blood pressure monitoring is useful to diagnose white-coat hypertension and non-dippers.
- Lifestyle modification aimed and modest weight reduction are effective.
- Total deaddiction is highly recommended in hypertensive diabetics.
- ACE inhibitors, beta-blockers, CCB and diuretics are commonly used agents to control hypertension.
- Clinical profile of individual patient dictates the choice of 1st drug to be employed for controlling blood pressure of a diabetic.

Chapter 19

# Dyslipidemia in Diabetes

It has been established beyond doubt that diabetics have a high risk of developing cardiovascular morbidity and mortality. One of the main risk factor for high CV complication is dyslipidemia. Many trials have shown that controlling dyslipidemia reduces CV risk considerably.

Typical dyslipidemia in diabetic person is raised triglycerides, low HDL high Apo-B and marginally raised LDL. However, LDL consists of small dense particles and is more atherogenic. Indians in particular have tendency to have very high triglyceride levels and low HDL levels.

## MECHANISM OF DIABETIC DYSLIPIDEMIA

Dyslipidemia in diabetics is the result of abnormal metabolism of lipoproteins, VLDL and HDL insulin resistance leads to excessive free fatty acid release from adipose tissues. Free fatty acids are converted into VLDL, TG and Apo-B. In normal person cholestreol ester transfer protein exchanges VLDL with HDL. HDL is broken down by hepatic lipase and then excreted in urine. In presence of excess VLDL there is increased exchange of HDL cholesterol for VLDL triglyceride. This leads to depletion of HDL.

## GOALS FOR THERAPY

- LDL should be below 100 mg% in patients with low CV risk.
- LDL should be below 70 mg% in patients with high CV risk.
- Triglyceride preferably below 150 mg%.
- HDL should be above 45 mg%.

## MANAGEMENT

- *Diet*: Low calorie diet with reduction in simple carbohydrates helps in improving dyslipidemia. Substitution of saturated fats by mono-unsaturated fats and reducing cholesterol containing food items helps a lot too. Use of fish, vegetables and legumes in larger proportion and less of animal fat is quite effective.
- Stopping alcohol intake results in reduction of triglycerides.
- Weight loss has been shown to be effective in improvement in dyslipidemia.
- Tight glycemic control by whatever means improves hypertriglyceridemia.
- *Lipid lowering drugs*: HMG CoA inhibitors (Statins), fibric acid derivatives, and bile acid binding resins, niacin are the main drugs, which are used to manage dyslipidemia. Other drugs like N3 fatty acids, cholesterol absorption inhibitors and hormone replacement therapy are used in selected cases. Let us see each group in more details.

A. *HMG CoA reductase inhibitors*: Commonly known as Statins- are very effective agents to reduce cholesterol. They act by competitively inhibiting the key enzyme HMG CoA, which is needed for a rate-limiting step of cholesterol synthesis. The main effect is on LDL cholesterol (Approx. 45-60%). There is some reduction in triglyceride level too, especially when the baseline values are high. Modest increase HDL is also seen with these agents.

Commonly used drugs are atorvastatin, simvastatin and rozuvastatin. Pravastatin is used less often. Main side effect of these agents is rhabdomylitis. Fortunately it is quite infrequent when these agents are used in sub maximal dosage. Some elevation in liver enzymes is seen with these agents. Various trials like 4-S, HPS, TNT, CARDS and Jupiter have shown significant benefits in CV morbidity and mortality with use of these agents. Usual dose of atorvastatin is 10-80 mg/day, simvastatin 5-20 mg/day and rozuvastatin 5-20 mg/day. Higher dose of statins are of particular use during acute coronary syndrome as they help in plaque stabilization.

B. Fibric acid derivatives (Fibrates) are peroxisome proliferator activated receptor $\alpha$ agonist. Commonly used agents are gemfibrozil and fenofibrate. They lower triglycerides by 35-50%, and raise HDL by 10-20%. The effect on LDL is variable. They act mainly by decreasing hepatic VLDL production and increasing fractional removal of VLDL triglyceride from plasma. Dose of gemfibrozil is 600 mg twice daily and that of fenofibrate is 145 mg/day. Side effects include some drug interactions as these agents have strong affinity for albumin. They are contraindicated in cases with gall stones.

   Various trials with fibrates (Helsinki heart study, VA – HDL intervention Trial, Field trial) can be referred to for effects of fibrates on LDL and overall cardiac benefits.

C. Niacin (nicotinic acid) is a very potent agent to reduce triglycerides and to raise HDL. It reduces hepatic VLDL production and increases synthesis of Apo A-1. Main problem with niacin is side effect, which include skin rash, flushes, acid peptic disease, hepatic dysfunction and alteration in glycemic control. Side effects are found to be relatively less with intermediate acting preparations of niacin. These are not easily available for routine use in patients with hypertriglyceridemia.

D. Ezitimibe is the latest and very effective agent, which reduces LDL by reducing cholesterol absorption from intestines. Dose is 10 mg per day. Reduction achieved in LDL is about 20% but impressive results are achieved when it is combined with statins.

E. Bile acid binding resins were used in past for reducing cholesterol. Agents include cholestyramine, colestipol and colesevelam. They get bound to bile acids in intestine and thus interrupt the enterohepatic re-circulation of bile acids. It results in decrease in amount of bile acids returning to liver and increased conversion of hepatic cholesterol to bile acids. As these drugs are to be taken in large volume, the compliance was low. They are also known to raise triglycerides in type 2 diabetics. Usage of these drugs has been markedly reduced after the availability of statins. Recent report of HbA1C reduction (0.4%) with use of colesevelam has created some new interest in this agent.

F. N3 fatty acids like decosa-hexanoic (DHA) and eicosapentanoic acid (EPA) when used in dose of 3-6 gm per day have resulted in significant reduction in triglyceride levels, especially when the levels are > 600 mg%. The question whether low dose of these molecules are effective in lowering triglycerides is unanswered.

G. Hormone replacement therapy with combination of estrogen and progesterone was said to reduce cardiovascular risk but recent results of HERS and WAVE trials tell us just the opposite. Hence, the benefit of hormone replacement therapy for cardiac benefits should be carefully evaluated in each case.

### Steps to be Taken for Treating Dyslipidemia in Diabetics

- Diet modification
- Regular exercise
- Stop alcohol
- Consider side effects of some drugs steroids, thiazide, rosiglitazone – replace them with a safer agent.
- High LDL – statins, ezitimibe, bile acid binding resins
- High triglyceride – fibrates, niacin, N3 fatty acids

The aim of therapy is to reduce CV risk in every diabetic person.

Choice of therapy as per lipid abnormality

| | *First choice* | *Second choice* | *Third choice* |
|---|---|---|---|
| High LDL | Statins | Bile acid binding resins | Fibrates |
| Low HDL | Lifestyle change | Niacin | Fibrates |
| High triglyceride | Glucose control | Fibrates | Statin in high dose |
| Mixed dyslipidemia | Glucose control and statins | Add fibrates | Replace fibrates by niacin |

Chapter 20

# Diabetic Foot

Foot problems in a diabetic person often take a disastrous course. They end in amputation and death of the person. These conditions are easily preventable if proper care is taken during the management of the patient. The underlying pathology is neuropathy—the condition that is asymptomatic in nearly 50% of the cases. Tobacco use, alcohol addiction, poverty, illiteracy, habit of walking barefoot, dyslipidemia and poor glycemic control are other contributory factors that lead to major foot problems in a diabetic person. Proper foot examination in a diabetic person will have great impact in preventing this complication.

Diabetic sensory neuropathy is usually symmetrical, progressing from distal to proximal areas. Numbness in limbs may be accompanied by hyperalgesia or hyperasthesia. Pain can be pricking or burning. It is more at night and is partly relieved by short walk. Intensity of pain may disturb sleep of the patient.

Sensory neuropathy is associated with motor weakness leading to weakness of small muscles of foot. There is alteration in normal alignment of tarsal bones. Unusually, high pressure points develop and then the person is more likely to develop ulcers from internal injury. External injury may go unnoticed and result delay in initiation of wound care. Foot problems after a religious tour (when person walks barefoot) or after a holiday on beach (sand particles enter through small cracks over-foot) are quite common and result in disastrous consequences.

Autonomic neuropathy accompanies many patients with peripheral neuropathy. It causes reduced sweating and more dryness of the skin. Cracks on sole are common in these patients. These cracks act as entry points for infection.

Various mechanisms like uncontrolled hyperglycemia, oxidative stress, nonenzymatic glycation, vascular factors, nerve growth factor anomalies, immunological alterations and polyol pathways are implicated in causation of diabetic neuropathy.

Age of the patient, degree of glycemic control, duration of diabetes, smoking, alcohol consumption, hypertension, dyslipidemia and presence of other microvascular complications of diabetes are risk factors for development of diabetic foot problem.

## EXAMINATION OF FOOT

- History
- Inspection
- Pulses
- Portable Doppler
- Monofilament test
- Joint mobility
- Motor functions

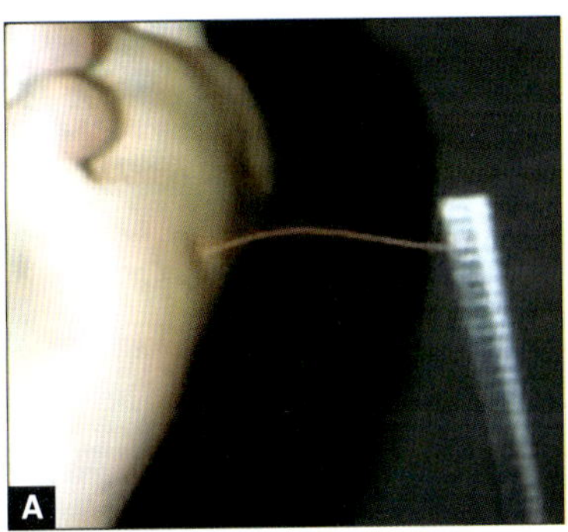

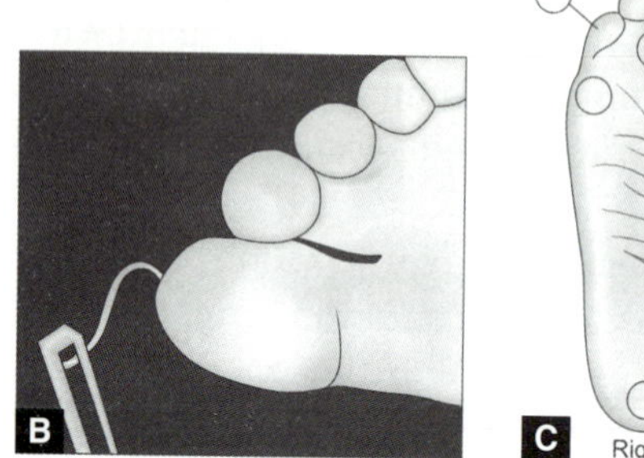

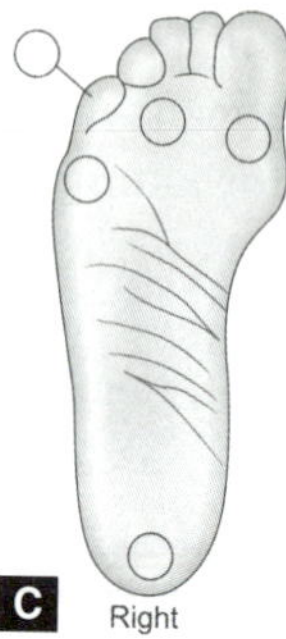

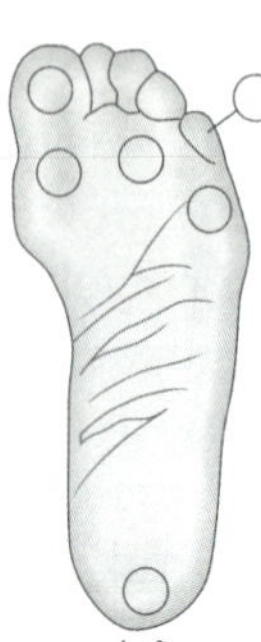


**Figures 20.1A to C:** Monofilament testing sites

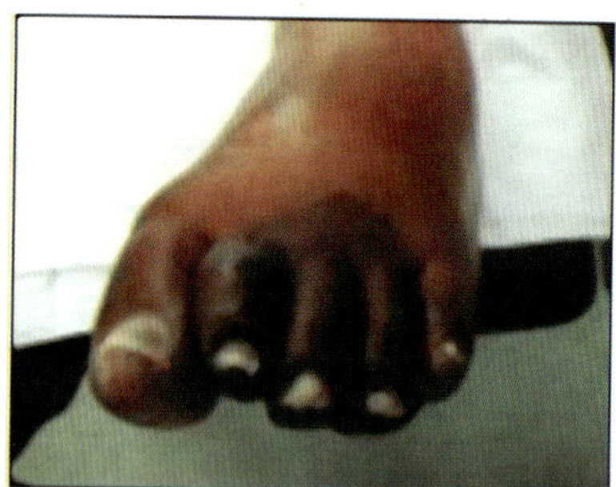

**Figure 20.2:** Foot gangrene

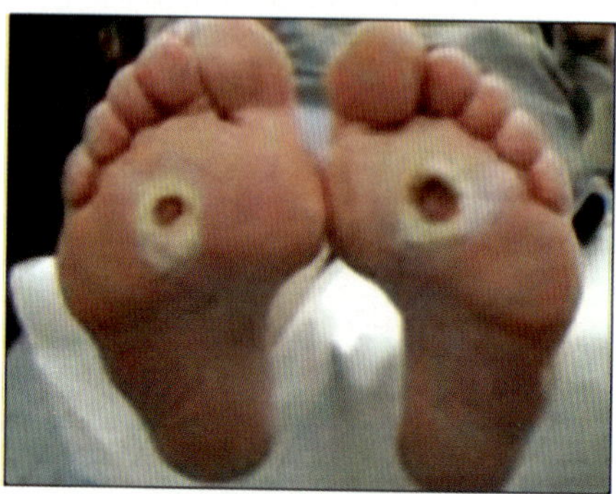

**Figure 20.3:** Foot ulcer

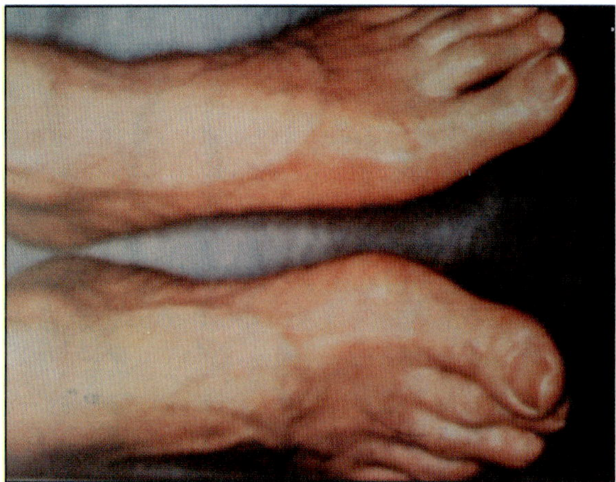

**Figure 20.4:** Prominent veins due to DAN

- Inspection—shape, skin color, ingrown toenail, prominent veins, ulcer or injury, swelling or redness of skin, foreign body.
- Inspection should be carried out in standing and lying down position to find deformities out of posture.
- Palpation for peripheral pulses, warmth, tenderness, foreign body, etc.
- Check for sensation using 10 gm monofilament, 128 Hz tuning fork at apex of hallux, pinprick and light sensation. Check for ankle jerk.
- Slow capillary and delayed venous filling suggest vascular insufficiency.
- Check for unsteadiness while standing and walking.
- Check footwear of the patient for asymmetrical wear and tear, foreign body like sand or small nail.

Use of an 8 MHz or 5 MHz Doppler probes is useful to assess vascular insufficiency when peripheral pulses are not palpable.

Ankle-brachial index must be calculated by measuring blood pressure at cubital fossa and at ankle. Ratio less than 1 indicates vascular insufficiency but one should be aware of false positive result in patients with severe atherosclerosis. Patients with vascular insufficiency give history of intermittent claudications and of tobacco use.

Biosthesiometer or vibratometer can be used to quantify vibration sensation. Normal threshold for vibratory perception is 15 volts.

Diabetic person can get neuropathy due to other causes like leprosy, alcohol, paramalignant syndrome, renal failure, hypothyroidism, nutritional deficiency or drug induced. One must be aware of these causes and try to rule out them before making a diagnosis of diabetic peripheral neuropathy.

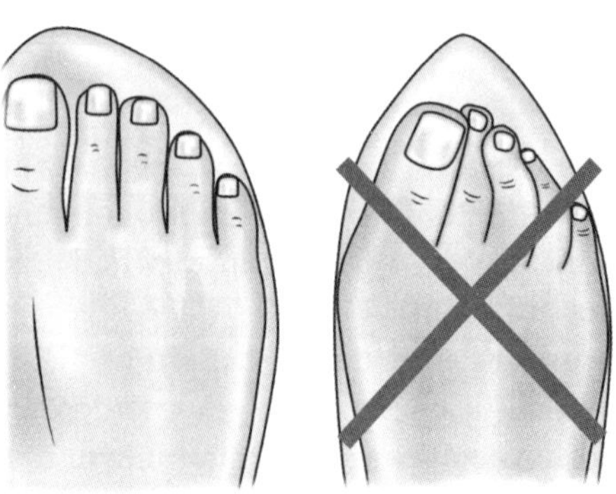

**Figure 20.5:** Not too tight footwear

## MANAGEMENT PRINCIPLES OF DIABETIC FOOT

- Early intervention.
- Aggressive surgical approach.
- Proper antibiotics
- Tight glucose control
- Say no to nicotine
- Health education
- Proper footwear

Proper steps taken at proper time by the patient and the treating physician will prevent amputation in large number of cases.

Chapter 21

# Eye Problems in Diabetes

One of the most studied organ in diabetes is eye. Studies like DCCT and UKPDS has shown that tight control of diabetes reduces incidence of retinopathy in type I and type II diabetics respectively. Eye disease in diabetes is usually associated with other microvascular complications like nephropathy and neuropathy. One can make use of dilated fundus examination to determine whether nephropathy is a diabetic person is due to diabetes or some other non-diabetic cause.

Various eye ailments, which occur in diabetes, are:

- Diabetic retinopathy—nonproliferative and proliferative macular edema.
- Cataract—early and rapidly progressive.
- Glaucoma—open angle and closed angle.
- Cranial nerve palsy affecting III, IV and VI.
- Early presbyopia.
- Recurrent conjunctivitis.
- Corneal abrasion.
- Fluctuating visual impairment.

Diabetic retinopathy (DR) is an important complication of diabetes, which if detected early and managed properly, can preserve vision.

It is classified into.

- Nonproliferative diabetic retinopathy (NPDR)
- Proliferative retinopathy.

Both of these conditions may or may not be associated with diabetic macular edema (DME).

Three stages of NPDR are:

- *Mild* with one or both of the following:
  - Few scattered retinal microaneurysms and hemorrhages
  - Hard exudates.

- *Moderate* with one or more of the following:
  - More extensive retinal microaneurysms and hemorrhages.
  - Mild intraretinal microvascular abnormalities (IRMA).
  - Early venous bleeding.
- *Severe NPDR* – one or more of the following:
  - Severe retinal microaneurysms and hemorrhages in all 4 quadrants.
  - Venous bleeding in at least two quadrants.
  - More extensive IRMA in at least one quadrant.
  - Proliferative diabetic retinopathy has got two stages.

*Early*

- Minimal ≤ 1/4th disk area—new vessels over disk (NVD) without preretinal or vitreous hemorrhage.
- New vessels elsewhere in retina (NVE) without hemorrhage.

*High-risk*

- NVD > 1/4th disk area without preretinal or vitreous hemorrhage.
- NVD < 1/4th disk area with fresh preretinal or vitreous hemorrhage.
- NVE > ½ disk area with preretinal or vitreous hemorrhage.

Status of macula is very important in diabetic eye disease as it can determine the course of visual loss. It can be assessed by slit-lamp examination, fundus photography or by latest method of ocular coherence tomography. There is collection of fluid over macula (Diabetic Macular Edema—DME) or there are hard exudates within macular area. Ophthalmic evaluation is needed to decide whether macular edema is clinically significant (CSME). Retinal thickening, hard exudates close to the disk and large lesions indicate CSME.

Risk factors for progression of DR are poor diabetes control, hypertension, kidney disease, hypercholesteremia, anemia, pregnancy, use of diuretics and duration of diabetes.

Every type II diabetic should have complete eye examination at the time of diagnosis and every year thereafter. For type I diabetics initial examination is done within 3-5 years of diagnosis or during puberty. Yearly follow-up is recommended for type I diabetics too. Eye examination should be carried out in diabetic women during childbearing age who are planning pregnancy, pre-conception then once or more frequently during each trimester and 6 weeks after delivery.

Staging of retinopathy determines the further examination schedule, investigations, treatment and prognosis.

| *Stage of retina* | *Follow-up in months* | *Fundus photography* | *Fluorescein angiography* | *Laser therapy* |
|---|---|---|---|---|
| Normal | 12 | No | No | No |
| Mild NDPR, No DME | 6-12 | Rarely | No | No |
| Moderate NDPR +DME | 4-6 | Occasionally | Rarely | No |
| NDPR + CSME | 2-4 | Yes | Yes | Yes |
| Severe NDPR | 2-4 | Yes | Yes if CSME | Consider |
| Early PDR | 2-4 | Yes | Yes if CSME | Consider |
| High-risk PDR | 2-4 | Yes | Yes if CSME | Yes |
| Unresponsive PDR | 1-4 | If possible | No | Yes, with vasectomy |

Treatment of high-risk PDR is done with full scatter laser. Around 1200 to 2000 lesions are applied to posterior pole in two or more sittings. Response to laser therapy is variable and at times unpredictable. Minor change in visual acuity and peripheral visual loss is seen in some cases after laser therapy.

CSME needs focal laser therapy. Aim of therapy is to halt further drop in visual acuity.

Newer modes of treatment like anti-VEGF agents or ruboxistaurin (Protein kinase–C inhibitor) are showing some promising results.

Patient with retinal detachment, nonresolving vitreous hemorrhage has to undergo to vitrectomy.

Other eye manifestations are discussed in brief.

## CATARACT

Cataract occurs more frequently in diabetics. It affects relatively younger people and progresses rapidly. Preoperative assessment of retinal status is useful to provide information about likely benefit after cataract surgery. Scatter laser therapy may be employed before cataract surgery in those with high-risk PDR. Implantable lens is preferred mode of surgery in this era.

Postoperative period is usually uneventful. At times closed angle glaucoma develops after cataract surgery. This is because of neovasularization over iris, local inflammation and fibrosis. It is called as neovasularization glaucoma (NVG). This is more likely to occur in patients with active PDR. Treatment of NVG is complicated and includes combination of laser, intraocular anti-VEGF agents, topical mydriatics or steroids, etc.

Person with uncontrolled diabetes will have reversible lenticular opacities. It can produce temporary problems in vision. They are corrected after stabilizing glucose levels.

## GLAUCOMA

Open angle glaucoma is twice more common is diabetics. Usual medical line of treatment is usually enough. Trabeculoplasty with argon-laser is needed in some cases.

Close angle glaucoma following cataract surgery is discussed above.

Cranial nerve paralysis occurs in diabetics, which leads to dipolpia. Sixth, fourth and third cranial nerves are commonly affected. These are called as noncompressive cranial nerve palsies as they are due to microinfarcts within the nerve fiber. Fibers that control size of the pupil are

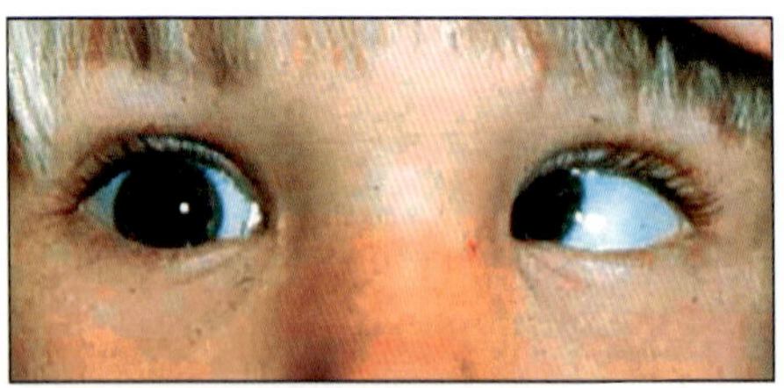

**Figure 21.1:** VI nerve palsy

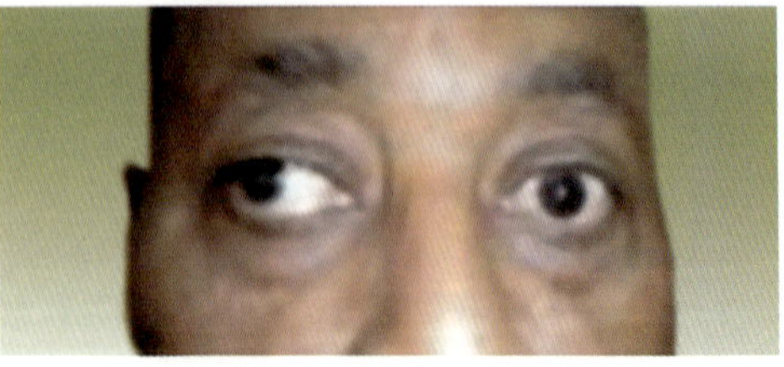

**Figure 21.2:** III nerve palsy

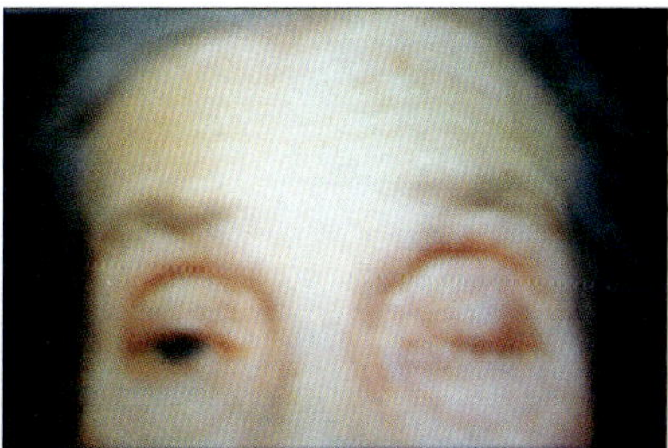

**Figure 21.3:** Ptosis

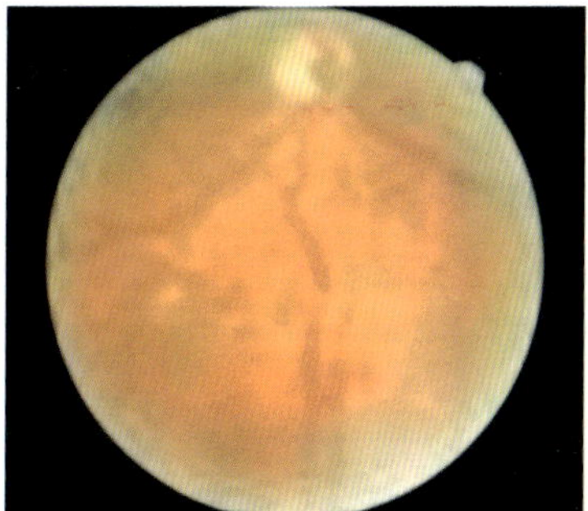

**Figure 21.4:** Early proliferative diabetic retinopathy

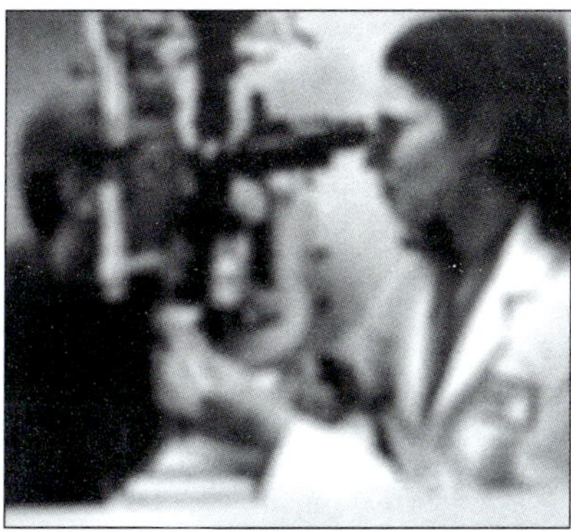

**Figure 21.5:** Eye check-up

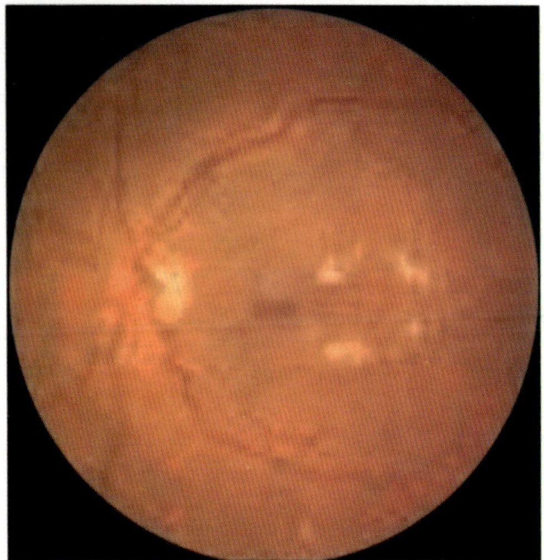

**Figure 21.6:** Nonproliferative diabetic retinopathy

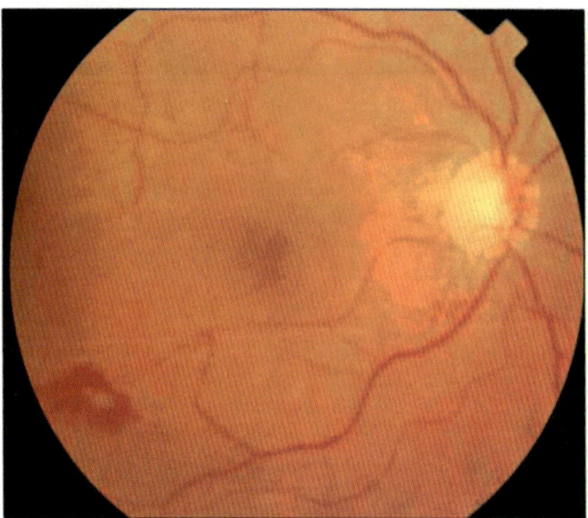

**Figure 21.7:** Proliferative diabetic retinopathy

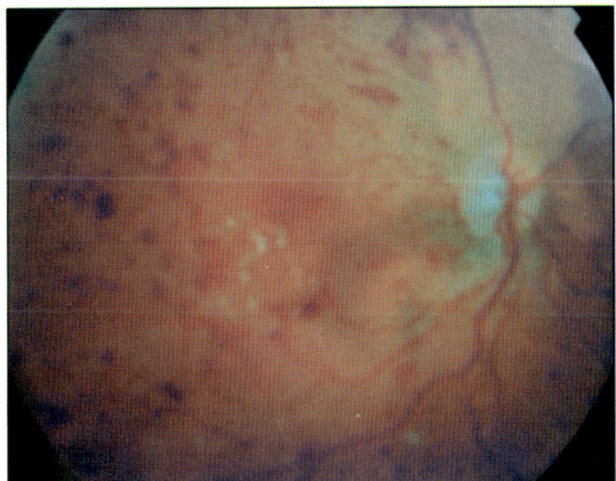

**Figure 21.8:** Severe retinal hemorrhage

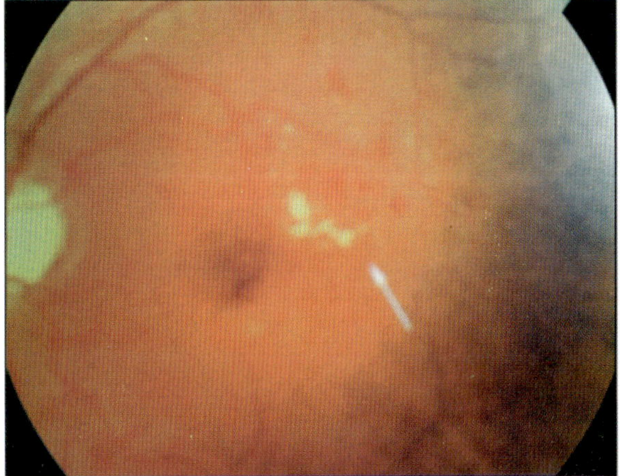

**Figure 21.9:** Severe form of retinal hemorrhage

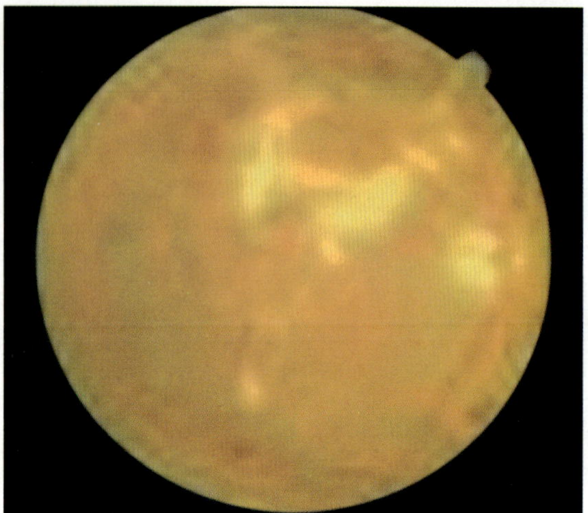

**Figure 21.10:** Severe PDR

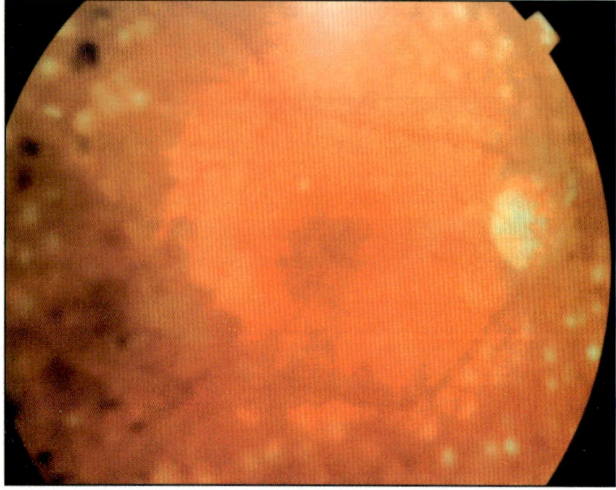

**Figure 21.11:** Severe retinal hemorrhage with laser scars

situated in the outermost layer of third cranial nerve. They are affected early in case of a lesion compressing third nerve, and are not affected in case of noncompressive third nerve palsy. Examination of pupil helps to decide about nature of third nerve palsy and thereby avoiding unnecessary and costly imaging studies of brain.

Yearly check-up of eyes of a diabetic person will lead to early detection of diabetic retinopathy. This will ensure timely treatment, which in turn will prevent blindness.

# Chapter 22

# Diabetic Nephropathy

Diabetes disturbs the function of kidneys in nearly 30% of cases. More than 10 million patients are suffering from this complication. The basic underlying pathology is micro-vascular disturbance. It is a major cause of morbidity and mortality in these cases. The natural course of the disease is similar in both type I and type II diabetics. Predictable course during early phase of this complication of diabetes is an unique feature. Subclinical stage of nephropathy is detected by checking urine for microalbuminuria. It is followed by stage of overt nephropathy during which progressive fall in glomerular filtration rate (GFR) is the rule. Rate of fall of GFR is variable. The range being 1-24 ml/min/year. End stage renal disease (ESRD) is the ultimate stage of diabetic nephropathy. Fortunately, good glycemic control can significantly decrease the development and rate of progression of diabetic nephropathy. This complication is usually associated with retinopathy and neuropathy as these too are microvascular complication. Some genetic predisposition is seen patients who develop DN.

## PATHOPHYSIOLOGY

Hyperglycemia, glycation products, growth factors, vasoactive hormones and cytokines, renal hemodynamic factors, hypertension, hyperlipidemia, smoking and few other factors play role in producing renal injury.

In a normal person 2 gm of albumin is filtered but most of it is re-absorbed by proximal tubules. If this reabsorbtion is inefficient then microalbuminuria sets in. As duration of diabetes increases, proteinuria goes up and GFR comes down. If untreated nearly 2/3rd of these cases will end up with ESRD.

## STAGES OF DIABETIC NEPHROPATHY

- Enlarged kidneys, high GFR, no symptoms.
- Normoalbuminuria (Albumin excretion rate (AER) < 30 mg/24 hrs).
- Incipient nephropathy AER 30-300 mg/24 hr, BP starts going up. This stage can be reversed or arrested by LSM and some medication.
- Overt diabetic nephropathy – Frank proteinuria, creatinine, BUN on the rise.
- ESRD–very low GFR needs renal replacement therapy.

Risk of rapid decline in GFR rises abruptly when HbA1C is steadily > 7.5% and PPBSL is persistently above 200 mg%.

## CLINICAL PRESENTATION

Patients are asymptomatic till the stage of over nephropathy. Episodes of hypoglycemia in a previously stable patient should alert a clinician about possibility of nephropathy, especially when the patient is on glibenclamide or metformin. Checking urine for micro-albuminuria can pick up incipient stage of nephropathy. Testing urine for sugar should now be replaced by testing for microalbuminuria. This simple test can be performed at any primary care physician or a family doctor. It needs no special equipment. What one needs is awareness!

Overt nephropathy and ESRD present with edema, shortness of breath, headache, nausea, anorexia, vomiting, hiccups, itching, anemia, blurred vision, etc. Patient may note frothiness in urine. Accelerated blood pressure is the rule. High dosage of multiple antihypertensive agents is needed to control blood pressure.

Tests like renal angiography, captopril scan and kidney biopsy are rarely needed to rule out nondiabetic cause of nephropathy.

## MANAGEMENT

- Tight control of blood glucose especially during early phase of diabetes by LSM, proper selection of anti-hyperglycemic agents is very important for long-term benefits.
- Protein restriction up to 0.8 gm/kg body weight is recommended. Use of class 1 proteins in these cases. Salt restriction is re-enforced. Small frequent feeds are advocated to prevent hypoglycemic. Fluid restriction is vital in case there is oliguria and fluid overload. Avoid glibenclamide, metformin and AGI. Insulin should be the drug of choice. Impaired insulin clearance and reduced renal gluconeogenesis increase the risk of hypoglycemia. On the other hand there is rise in insulin resistance. Hence, fluctuating blood glucose levels is quite common in patients with ESRD. Short acting insulin analogues are preferred agents as they have predictable action profile even with rising doses, less risk of hypoglycemia.
- Blood pressure control by judicious use of various anti-hypertensive drugs acting at different sites is needed. Potassium sparing diuretics are best avoided. Postural hypotension must be specifically looked for and then managed. Target BP is 130/80 in patients without albuminuria and 125/75 in those with albuminuria. ACEI, ARB, CCB, diuretics are preferred agents.

- Take care of hyperkalemia, hyperphosphatemia and hypocalcemia.
- Anemia is to be corrected by Inj. erythropoetin, PCV and hematinics.
- Acidosis is managed by soda-bicarb and diet modification.
- Diuretics are needed for those with signs of CHF.
- Hypoprotenemia is corrected by supplementing IV amino acids and by reducing protein loss with ACEI, ARB, amlodipine, atorvastatin, and pentoxyfylline, etc. Assess cardiac status of every patient with DN.
- Look for and treat associated microvascular complications like retinopathy, neuropathy.
- Newer drugs like aliskiren (Renin blocker), ruboxistaurin (Protein kinase-C inhibitor), pyridoxamin.
- Stop tobacco in all forms like smoking, chewing, intranasal and, gingival route.
- Renal replacement therapy:
  - Dialysis (Hemo or peritoneal)
  - Renal transplant.

Hemodialysis is initially carried out through a femoral or radial catheter. Later on an arteriovenous fistula is created in order to have quick and easy access to bloodstream. Usual frequency of hemodialysis is 3 times a week. It is an outpatient procedure and time needed for one sitting is 4 hrs. Procedure is slower than hemodialysis.

Peritoneal dialysis involves transportation of dialysis solution into abdominal cavity through a permanently placed catheter. It collects waste products and excess water from peritoneal blood vessels. The solution is then drained out of abdomen. The procedure slower than hemodialysis.

It carries risk of infection in diabetic patients. Patient at his home can perform this type of dialysis after proper training.

By law renal transplantation can be performed in diabetic person provided donor is a close relative of the patient. The donor's kidney should be matched to recipient by blood type, HLA type and cross matching antigens. Cadaveric renal transplant is not so popular in our country. Combined renal and pancreatic transplantation has shown better results than renal transplant alone.

## SUMMARY

- Diabetic nephropathy affects 30% of diabetics.
- Early detection of asymptomatic and reversible stage is possible by a simple test like checking urine for microalbuminuria.
- ACEI and other drugs can revert the progression of nephropathy.
- Dialysis can be postponed by intensive medical line of treatment if it started early.
- Renal replacement therapy is a must for ESRD.

Chapter 23

# Autonomic Neuropathy and Diabetes

Diabetics who have genetic predisposition to develop classical diabetic peripheral neuropathy go through a long silent phase before they have clinical symptoms. Many of them do have features of autonomic neuropathy too. These people can be picked up by complex electrophysiological studies or by simple clinical tests carried out by a smart clinician. Once autonomic neuropathy sets in, it progresses relentlessly to produce various clinical problems in a diabetic person. Hence, early recognition is quite important.

Cardiac, genitourinary and GI tract are the main systems, which are affected by autonomic neuropathy. Hypoglycemic unawareness is common in patients with autonomic neuropathy. Other less important effects are disturbances in sweating (more sweating in central areas, less in distal areas) and failure of papillary response to darkness.

Many cases with autonomic neuropathy have peripheral neuropathy, nephropathy and proliferative retinopathy. But not all patients with diabetic peripheral neuropathy have associated autonomic neuropathy.

Diabetic autonomic neuropathy (DAN) is usually asymptomatic or may present with silent. Postural vertigo, brittle diabetes due to gastroparesis or hypoglycemia unawareness. Steno 2 study has shown that intensive control in type 2 diabetes results in slowing the progression of DAN.

Three stages of DAN are:

- Asymptomatic
- Abnormal autonomic testing
- Symptomatic.

Tests for autonomic neuropathy are:

- Heart rate variability on deep inspiration.
- Valsalva ratio.
- Postural drop in blood pressure by 20 mm.
- Nuclear medicine studies for gastric motility.
- Urodynamic study.

## CLINICAL FEATURES OF DAN

### Cardiovascular

- Resting tachycardia due to lack of vagal tone
- Exercise intolerance
- Higher prevalence of CHF
- Intraoperative CV instability – Hypotension and arrhythmia
- Increased mortality after AMI
- Sudden death due to arrhythmia
- Orthostatic hypotension due to lack of vasoconstriction in splanchnic and peripheral circulation.

It can lead to dizziness, falls, fractures and loss of sensorium. It increases the risk of diabetic nephropathy and stroke. It is more common in postprandial period. It is associated with normal diurnal variation in blood pressure. Antihypertensive drugs and antidepressnats aggravate postural hypotension. Hence, while managing patient with DAN try to look for a treatable cause. Sitting and standing should be a slow process in people with DAN. Elevation of head by 30 cm above the bed is of doubtful benefit. Body stocking is of some value. Drugs used for postural hypotension are fludrocortisone, fluoxetine, midodrine, erythropoetin, desmopressin, pindolol and octerotide, etc. Overall response to drug therapy is far from optimal.

### DAN and Genitourinary System

Main problems arising out of DAN in relation to GU system are:

- Erectile dysfunction (ED)
- Retrograde ejaculation
- Bladder dysfunction
- Dyspareunia in females

#### *Erectile Dysfunction (ED)*

Erectile dysfunction (ED) is present in nearly 50 % of patients with long standing, i.e. more than 10 years of diabetes. Rarely, it can be the presenting symptom of diabetes. History taking of all male diabetics should include a question or two about his sexual activity. The etiology of ED in diabetics is complex. It includes vascular and neurogenic factors. At times there are some psychological factors too.

Onset of ED is usually insidious but may be abrupt in some cases. Psychological factors may play important role at this juncture. Usual presenting feature at onset is lack of hardness to achieve penetration or inability to maintain erection till ejaculation. Rarely, other causes of ED like low testosterone or hyperprolactinemia are also present in diabetics. Some medications like antihypertensive or anti-depressants or tranquilizers can contribute to ED to some extent. History of nitrate use must be asked as these patients will be given sildenafil.

Morning erections which take place for more than 3 times a week indicates psychogenic factors. At times stamp-test is needed to assess nocturnal tumescence. In patients with ED libido is usually normal.

### Treatment of ED

Invention of phosphodiesterase 5 inhibitors (PDEF) have revolutionized treatment of ED. Three molecules are available from this group... Sildenafil, tadanafil and verdanafil. They differ in duration of action. Sildenafil acts for 24 hrs while tadanafil acts for about 72 hrs. These drugs should be taken after food in order to minimize esophagitis. After oral administration the onset of action is seen after 30 minutes. Patient and his partner should be informed about this in order to achieve desired results. Usual drug of 1st choice is sildenafil. One starts with 25 mg dose and the maximum dose is 100 mg. Side effects include headache, altered perception of blue color and esophagitis. One can combine sildenafil with either verdanafil or tadanafil when sildenafil alone fails. If the combination fails then look for other causes of ED like hypogonadism.

Other forms of treatment for ED include intracavernosal injection of phenotalmine, intraurethral alprostadil, vacuum therapy and penile prosthesis. These are rarely needed in this era of PDEF inhibitors.

#### *Retrograde Ejaculation*

Retrograde ejaculation is the result of DAN, which leads to in coordination of bladder sphincters. This can result in infertility. Urine is cloudy and urine-analysis shows sperms. Ant-histaminic are found to be of some use in these cases.

#### *Bladder Dysfunction*

Bladder dysfunction results due to bladder denervation. Patients do not have sensation of full bladder. The frequency of urination drops down to some extent. Incomplete emptying of bladder is the rule. Residual urine leads to recurrent urinary tract infections. At times retention with overflow takes place.

It can be managed by timed urination, intermittent self-catheterization and by using bethanechol 10-30 mg /day.

### *Dyspareunia*

Dyspareunia is common in diabetic women. One of the cause for it is decreased lubrication as a result of DAN. Other causes are hormonal deficiency and monilial infection. Treatment of last two causes by hormone replacement and antimonilial agents corrects the problem. PAP smear is recommended for patients with recurrent or chronic vaginitis.

## Gastrointestinal Tract and DAN

### *Esophageal Dysmotility*

Esophageal dysmotility, gastroparesis and diabetic diarrhea are main features of DAN.

Esophageal dysmotility leads to dysphagia, heartburn and retrosternal pain. Treatment is domperidone.

### *Gastroparesis*

Gastroparesis is known to occur in patients with long standing diabetes. It results in upper abdominal discomfort and fullness. Nausea, anorexia and at times vomiting. They have high-risk of aspiration pneumonia while recovering from anesthesia.

Gastroparesis can cause irregular absorption of oral hypoglycemic agents. It can lead to "brittle " diabetes.

Diagnosis of gastroparesis is made by upper GI endoscopy. Isotope studies are expensive and rarely needed.

Treatment of gastroparesis is frequent small feeds with liquid diet. Drugs like metochopropamide, domperidone, Cisapride are useful but tachyphylaxis and other side effects are troublesome in some patients. Erythromycin in suspension form is found to be of some use.

Exanatide and pramlintide are avoided in patients with gastroparesis. Rapid acting insulin analogues are contraindicated in these patients. At times, it is advisable to give insulin at the end of the meal in order to achieve good postmeal glucose control. Very rarely surgical approach is used for jejunal feeding or for implanting a gastric pacemaker.

#### *Diabetic Diarrhea*

Nocturnal painless liquid diarrhea is main characteristic features of diabetic diarrhea. The cause of this problem is intestinal bacterial overgrowth. Tropical pancreatitis and celiac disease are other causes of diarrhea in diabetic person in tropical countries and in caucasian population respectively.

Treatment includes tetracycline, loperamide, and lomotil and in some cases injection octreotide. Metformin is to be avoided in these cases. Dietary changes may me tried but overall response to therapy is far from satisfactory.

Overall DAN is relatively neglected yet very important area of diabetes management. Little attention to persistent complaints like fluctuating glucose levels despite regular lifestyle and unaltered drug dose, or recurrent urinary tract infections, should alert a clinician about possibility of associated DAN. Simple clinical tests should establish the diagnosis. Additional treatment of DAN helps in getting steady glucose level.

Chapter 24

# Acute Myocardial Infarction in Diabetes

Diabetics are more susceptible to suffer from myocardial infarction as compared to nondiabetics. Acute myocardial infarction is the cause of death in nearly 50% of diabetics. The event takes place in relatively younger age group. The severity of acute coronary insufficiency is more in diabetics and so are the chances of reinfarction and congestive heart failure. Silent infarct is known nearly 1/3rd of diabetics who suffer from acute myocardial infarction. Even in symptomatic individuals, the symptoms may be nonspecific and vague. These facts underline the importance of high index of suspicion to have timely diagnosis.

Contributory factors for unfavorable outcomes are:

- Accelerated atherosclerosis
- Prothrombotic state
- Autonomic neuropathy → arrhythmia, hypotension
- Larger MI zone due to micro- and macrovascular disease
- Smoking.

## DIAGNOSIS

Diagnosis is made by:

- Classical symptoms of ischemia
- ECG showing fresh ischemia or Q waves
- Rise in CPK-MB, S GOT (S AST) or troponin level
- New regional wall motion abnormality on echo
- New loss of viable myocardium on perfusion scan.

## TREATMENT

Tight glucose control with insulin is a must for all patients with acute myocardial infarction.

### For ST Elevation Myocardial Infarction

- Fibrinolytic therapy with streptokinase or urokinase Or with alteplase or reteplase with heparin.
- Primary percutaneous intervention (PCI) with angioplasty in case the patient reaches early (within 60 minutes of presentation).
- Aspirin 325 mg per day.
- Clopidogrel 300 mg loading dose then 75 mg per day.
- Heparin – UFH or LMWH.
- Statins for plaque stabilization.

### For Non ST Elevation Myocardial Infarction

- Emergency primary PCI.
- Enoxaparin – a LMWH or GP IIa/IIIb inhibitors.
- Drug eluting stent (DES) or bare metal stent (BMS).
- Statins in high dose 40-80 mg of atorvastatin.
- ACE inhibitors or carvedilol in low dose.

## SURGERY FOR AMI IN DIABETES

Revascularization using internal mammary artery graft is preferred method over multiple stents, in diabetic patient with multivessel disease. Minimally, invasive surgical techniques are more useful in diabetics as they have faster and smoother postoperative recovery.

## LONG-TERM CARE AFTER A CORONARY EVENT

- Aspirin—162 to 325 mg per day for 1 month in patients with BMS—for 3-6 months in DES patients—75 to 150 mg day life-long

- Clopidogrel with or without aspirin, for one year
- Omit clopidogrel for 5-7 days before CABG
- Statins for lowering LDL below 100 mg%
- Fibrates for lowering triglycerides below 150 mg%
- Fibrates to raise HDL above 40 mg%
- Beta-blockers, preferably cardioselective
- ACE inhibitors – Ramipril
- Nitrates – long acting preparations.
  - Sublingual or spray for immediate relief
- Rehabilitation.

Successful outcome after acute myocardial infarction in a diabetic patient depends on proper metabolic control, prompt revascularization and adequate hemodynamic support. Although the prognosis is guarded in diabetic patients with acute myocardial infarction, early treatment within first hour at coronary care unit makes all the difference. With rising number of young patients with acute coronary insufficiency, there is undisputed need for more and more coronary care units in our country.

# Chapter 25

# Cardiac Evaluation in a Diabetic Person

Diabetics carry four fold more risk of developing ischemic heart disease as compared to nondiabetics. Diabetic women have more risk as compared to diabetic men. Prognosis is poor in diabetic population after acute coronary event. Results of revascularization are inferior in diabetics as opposed to those obtained in nondiabetics. Moreover coronary disease strikes early in diabetic patient. The risk is higher in those who use tobacco in any form and those who have one or more components of metabolic syndrome. Coronary artery disease is a major cause of death in diabetics. In fact diabetes has been labeled as independent risk factor for ischemic heart disease.

As the problem remains silent in most of the cases, high index of suspicion and routine testing for cardiac involvement is mandatory in order to pick-up the disease at early stage. Simple clinical tests can be combined with sophisticated investigations to yield the best results.

Clinical means like pulse, blood pressure, ankle-brachial index, signs of congestive cardiac failure (CCF) are of useful in gathering some basic information about cardiac status. Resting tachycardia, marked variability in heart rate with valsalva maneuver, hypertension, postural hypotension, low ankle-brachial index (A-B index), pallor, signs of CCF definitely indicate cardiac involvement. One should be careful while interpreting results of A-B index in an old person with calcification of vessels.

Checking urine for microalbuminuria provides additional information about endothelial dysfunction. Positive test for microalbuminuria is an independent risk factor for coronary heart disease.

Intima-medial thickness (IMT) is considered as a surrogate marker of atherosclerosis. Hence, carotid artery Doppler will give us some information about degree of atherosclerosis.

## INVESTIGATIONS

Investigations that are made use of to diagnose cardiac function in a diabetic person.

- Electrocardiogram (ECG)
- 2 D echocardiogram
- Tread mill test or computerized stress test
- Stress echocardiography
- Coronary angiography
- Cardiac perfusion studies.

### Electrocardiogram (ECG)

Basic investigation for cardiac assessment is 12 lead resting electrocardiogram (ECG) for detecting left ventricular hypertrophy, silent infarct, ST-T changes suggestive of ischemia and bundle branch blocks. Comparison with a previous ECG is often helpful to detect new events. But ECG has got some limitations like high rate of false negative results.

Therefore, further tests like 2 D echocardiogram (2 D ECHO) and computerized stress test (CST) are needed in many cases.

### 2 D Echocardiogram

This investigation gives information about left ventricular ejection fraction, ventricular wall thickness and wall motion abnormality. It gives information about status of cardiac valves, right ventricular function and pulmonary artery pressure too. Thrombus in the cardiac cavity might come as a surprise. Cardiomyopathy can be easily diagnosed with 2 D echo.

### Tread Mill Test or Computerized Stress Test

This test is performed to confirm the diagnosis of cardiac ischemia. Person is asked to run on a moving belt, the speed and inclination of which is gradually increased till the patient attains 85 % of his target heart rate (220 minus age in years). Horizontal or down-sloping ST segment depression for more than 1 mm at 60-80 mseconds beyond J point, occurring during exercise or during recovery period is interpreted as positive test for exercise induced ischemia.

At times CST has to stopped prematurely due to:

- More than 2 mm ST segment depression
- Fresh ST segment elevation without Q waves
- Drop in systolic blood pressure
- Absence of rise in systolic blood pressure after beginning the test
- Severe angina
- Ischemic changes within 3 minutes of staring the test
- Multifocal ventricular premature contractions.

CST can be false positive in patients with left ventricular hypertrophy and in female subjects.

Obesity, severe osteoarthritis, severe neuropathy and peripheral vascular disease are the conditions in which it is not possible to perform CST.

### Stress Echocardiography

Person is administered dobutamine and cardiac function is studied with echocardiography machine. Wall motion abnormality can precede classic angina in diabetics. Biphasic response or inability to increase contractility after dobutamine is suggestive of underlying ischemia. This test helps in distinguishing between hibernating, stunned or infracted myocardium.

### Coronary Angiography

When CST or stress ECHO reports indicate ischemic heart disease, coronary angiography is carried out. This procedure can be done either from femoral or radial artery under local

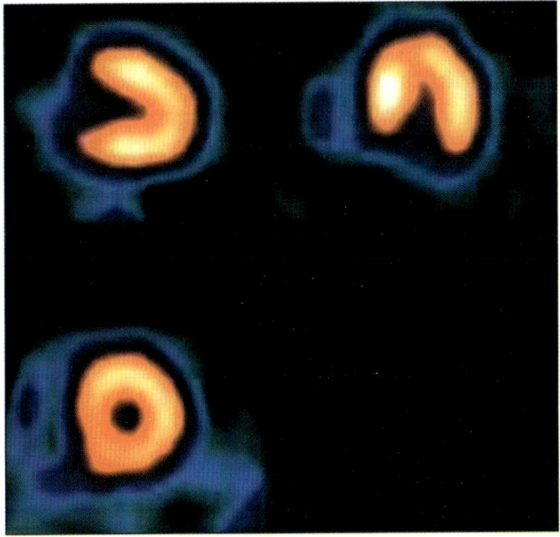

**Figure 25.1:** Thallium scan

anesthesia. Usual hospital stay is 6-8 hours. Ant platelet agents, aspirin and heparin have to be stopped for minimum 24 hours prior to the procedure. Degree and location of vascular block can be judged after studying the recording of the test. Person should be off metformin prior to angiography. The procedure carries a small risk of bleeding or infection at the site of vascular access, stroke, renal failure and myocardial infarction.

### Cardiac Perfusion Study

Patients who are not willing to undergo angiography can be evaluated by some advanced technological methods. These include myocardial perfusion studies (Single Photon Emission Computed Tomography—SPECT), Positron Emission Tomography (PET scan), Electron Beam Computed Tomography (EBCT), Multislice Computed Tomography coronary angiography (Coronary CT). Role of magnetic resonance angiography is yet to be established.

More *details of these investigations can be found in Appendix III.*

Chapter 26

# Infections in Diabetes

Diabetic patients are more likely to succumb to infections. They have reduced motility of phagocytes, which results in delay in entrapment of pathogenic organism. Raised blood sugar and acidic medium provide favorable conditions for growth of certain fungal pathogens that are specifically observed in diabetics.

Autonomic neuropathy leads to altered foot-mechanics, and the foot becomes more vulnerable to internal and external injury. Interruption of physical barrier of skin because of such injuries provides easy access to organisms into the body. Vascular insufficiency plays additional role in foot infections in diabetic person. Autonomic neuropathy leads to incomplete evacuation of bladder, which leads to recurrent urinary tract infections. Impaired cough reflex due to cerebrovascular insufficiency make the person more prone to develop pneumonia. Some changes in cell mediated immunity makes these patients more prone to chronic infections like tuberculosis.

Infections in a diabetic person are more severe and more widespread as compared to nondiabetic one. Moreover minor infection can progress to septicemia when there is uncontrolled hyperglycemia. On the other hand tight control of blood glucose with insulin leads to reduction in deaths due to septic shock. Good metabolic control improves outcome especially in surgical intensive care unit.

Some infections, which are specifically important in a diabetic, are discussed below.

## URINARY TRACT INFECTIONS

Asymptomatic bacteriuria is common especially in female diabetic patients. Cystitis, pyelonephritis and perinephric abscess are common in diabetics. Causative organisms are *E. coli*; Acute uncomplicated urinary tract infections can be managed by oral quinolones (Levofloxacin or moxifloxacin) or with trimethoprim-sufamethoxazole or with ampicillin plus clavulanate.

Hospitalization and intravenous antibiotic therapy is needed when the infection is not responding to oral antibiotics. They are managed by cefotaxime, ceftriaxone, or ticarcillin + clavulanate or piperacillin plus tazobactum combination. Some case may respond to vancomycin or nafcillin. Antibiotic therapy is continued for 14 days.

Investigations like ultrasonography, urine culture sensitivity tests and urodynamic studies should be used to find out underlying reason for poor response to treatment.

Balanitis and candidial vaginitis are common in diabetic patients. It can be a presenting symptom of diabetes in some cases. Response to fluconazole is satisfactory in most of the cases.

## FOOT INFECTIONS

Diabetic patient can get recurrent trauma to foot, which is not noticed immediately due to underlying neuropathy.

Foot infection, which is in the form of shallow ulcer, which is associated with minimal cellulitis and no tissue necrosis or systemic symptoms, is considered as non-limb threatening infection. Causative organisms are group A streptococci and *S. aureus*. Wound care and oral antibiotics are usually sufficient to control the problem. Clindamycin and amoxycilin + clavulanate or cephalexin is usual choice.

Infection that has spread into deeper planes and has caused significant tissue necrosis and systemic symptoms is considered as limb threatening infection. Causative organisms are gram-positive cocci, *E. coli*, *P. aeurigenosa* and anerobic bacteria. They need more aggressive management like surgical debridement and intravenous antibiotics. Higher antibiotics like ticarcillin + clavulanate or piperacillin plus tazobactum combination or imipenem + cilastatin are needed to control infection and save the limb.

Narcotizing gangrenous fascitis is peculiarly seen in diabetics. The causative organism is a betahemolytic *Streptococcus* or at times it could be polymicrobial. Treatment is same as that employed for limb threatening foot infections. Immunoglobulis and high dose may be of use when this condition is leading towards septic shock.

## LUNG INFECTIONS

Pulmonary tuberculosis is an important lung infection in diabetes. These patients are more prone to get widespread pulmonary lesions especially when the metabolic control is suboptimal. They are more likely to develop multidrug resistant tuberculosis (MDR Tb). Diabetes has to be managed with insulin when there is concomitant tuberculosis. Antitubercular treatment will last for longer duration in these cases.

Impaired cough reflex in diabetics with cerebrovascular insufficiency make them prone to get pneumonia. Organism like *Klebsiella*, *E. coli*, *Legionella*, Streptococci, *Aspergilus*, Mucor and Influenza virus are more likely to cause pneumonia in diabetics. Morbidity and mortality due to pneumonia is high in diabetics. Therefore, it is recommended that all diabetics should be vaccinated once with pneumococcal vaccine and with influenza vaccine one a year.

## ABDOMINAL INFECTIONS

Cholecystitis, typically emphysematous type, is more common in diabetics. It carries high mortality unless immediate surgical intervention with use of broad-spectrum antibiotics (Piperacillin + tazobactum or ceftazideine + metronidazole) is used.

Intestinal tuberculosis is more common in diabetics. Presetting features include low-grade fever, altered bowel movements, abdominal pain; weight loss and lump in right iliac fossa. Barium meal study or laparoscopy is diagnostic.

## MALIGNANT OTITIS EXTERNA

Malignant otitis externa is typically seen only in diabetics. The causative organism is *P. aurigenosa*. It starts as a chronic erosive process involving cartilage and soft tissues of external ear which progresses to involve petrous bone, temporal bone and mastoid. Further progression leads to lower cranial nerve palsy. Pain and purulent discharge are presenting features. Antibiotics like ciprofloxacin, ceftazidine, imipenem + cilastatin, meropenem, piperacillin are to be given for prolonged period along with bold surgical drainage.

## MUCORMYCOSIS

Mucormycosis is the worst infection faced by diabetic patient. It carries very high mortality. It is common in uncontrolled diabetes with ketoacidosis. Hyperglycemia and acidic medium provides best medium for growth of mycelia of fungi like mucor. They cause a fulminant necrotizing process, which involves nasal septum, para-nasal sinuses and orbit. Within few days the infection spreads to central nervous system. Early diagnosis with the help of deep surgical biopsy from necrosed area is the key to success. Differential diagnosis is aspergillosis. Proper and quick control of metabolic derangements, bold and repeated surgical intervention and amphoterecin B as ant-fungal agent may provide some hope to these patients.

## SKIN INFECTIONS

Skin infections are very common and recurrent in diabetics. It could be presenting feature in some cases. Usual sites are

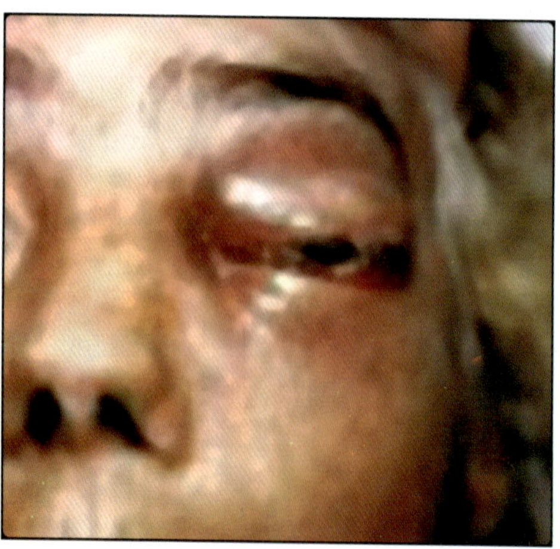

**Figure 26.1:** Mucormycosis

nape of the neck, armpit, inguinal region or genitals. The causative organisms are *S. aureus*, *Trichomonas* or *Candida*. In some cases the infection reaches deeper layers of skin, leading to abscess formation. Aggressive surgical drainage is needed in such cases.

A diabetic person can have catastrophic consequences after bacterial or fungal infections. This is particularly true in case of uncontrolled diabetics. Good metabolic control, use of higher antibiotics in adequate dosage and for sufficient duration, along with help of our surgical colleague will save life of our diabetic patient.

Chapter 27

# Skin Manifestations in Diabetics

Diabetes is a silent disease. Paucity of symptoms is characteristic aspect of this disease. The organ that is readily visible to the patient is of course skin. Hence, cutaneous manifestations in diabetes are important because they are helpful in early diagnosis of this disease.

Skin manifestations seen in a diabetic person could be either of the following type.

- Caused by metabolic derangements of diabetes
- Associated with diabetes
- Related to therapy
- Infections peculiar to diabetes
- Higher incidence in diabetes

## CAUSED BY METABOLIC ALTERATIONS OF DIABETES

- *Xanthoma and Xanthelamas*—due to hypercholesteremia
- Eruptive xanthomas
- *Carotinodermia*—in chronic uncontrolled diabetics.
- Acanthosis nigricans consists of velvety, brownish – black lesions, especially on back of neck, axilla, elbows, knuckles, perineal area, back of knee and dorsum of toes. They are bilaterally symmetrical. They are due to chronic insulin resistance, and therefore they are seen in patients with metabolic syndrome, PCOD or with obesity.

## ASSOCIATED WITH DIABETES

- Necrobiosis Lipoidica Diabeticorum (NLD)
- Lipodystrophies
- Diabetic dermopathy – Brown spots
- Glucagonoma syndrome
- Palmar sclerosis

- Bullosis diabeticorum
- Scleroderma diabeticorum

### Necrobiosis Lipoidica Diabeticorum (NLD)

- Etiology—unknown
- More common in type I cases
- More common in females, more in white race
- Age of presentation 30-50 years
- Bilaterally asymmetrical
- Starts as a small, well-demarcated, reddish papule.
- Changes into an atrophic plaque with raised borders and depressed center.
- Usual sites are anterior aspect of le, abdominal wall and arms
- Asymptomatic as long as there is no infection.
- May have atypical presentation like nodular or sclerodermatic
- Treatment—Protective skin pads
  - Occlusive steroid dressings
  - Intradermal steroids
  - Aspirin
  - Skin grafts

### Lipodystrophies

- Congenital or acquired
- Partial lipodystrophy
- Abnormal adipose distribution
  - Android (Upper body)- PCOD, HIV treatment
  - Lower body (Gynoid)

- Lipoatrophic diabetes
  - Severe insulin resistance, low leptin
  - But ketosis resistant
  - No subcutaneous fat
  - Acanthosis nigricans and skin tags are common
  - Dyslipidemia very common
  - Fatty liver, cirrhosis with portal hypertension
  - Thick bones
  - Muscular hypertrophy
  - Proteinuria common
  - Treatment – insulin, leptin and IGF

### Diabetic Dermopathy

- Most frequent dermopathy in diabetes.
- Small < 1 cm in size, brownish metallic in color
- Very common in men
- Anterior aspect of leg
- Age 60 years and above
- Usually associated with neuropathy or peripheral vascular disease.
- Can occur in non-diabetics too
- Less melanin and more hemosiderin is the cause.

### Glucagonoma Syndrome

- Common in mild diabetics or during IGT
- Necrotising migratory erythema is common
- Glossitis, stomatitis, vaginitis and brittle nails with weight loss are common associated features. Anemia, low serum proteins and high ESR are common too.

- High serum glucagon levels > 500 pgm/ml is diagnostic.
- High proglucagon percentage is noted. May secrete insulin, VIP or gastrin
- Eighty percent are malignant with high chance of metastasis in liver, spine, duodenum at the time of diagnosis.
- CT, MRI or angiography useful prior to surgery.
- Treatment includes surgery, replacement of amino acids by hyperalimentation, embolization of liver metastasis and somatostatin analogs.

### Palmar Sclerosis

- Also called as limited joint mobility syndrome or diabetic hand syndrome
- There is limited extension of metacorpo-phalyngeal joints, which leads to a small gap when patient is asked press to hands on each other, say while saying *NAMASTE*.

Hyperglycemia leads to glycation of proteins, followed by glycation of collagen. Increased cross linkage of collagen fibers leads to thickened, less digestible collagen fibers. Thick collagen results in thick skin in palmar aspect of hands and fingers. This leads to limited joint mobility.

It can remain asymptomatic in many cases. Nearly 15% of diabetics have some degree of palmar sclerosis. It is more common in uncontrolled and long standing diabetics. When a person places his hand on a flat surface, fanning of fingers is seen. Prominent flexor tendons are seen due to limited finger extension. The condition is associated with collagen vascular diseases and osteoarthritis. The condition improves with control of hyperglycemia.

## SKIN LESIONS DUE TO TREATMENT

SU group of drugs can cause allergic rash over skin. In previous days when chlorpropamide was available, severe flush after consumption of alcohol was observed in patients who were on this drug.

Insulin lipoatrophy or lipohypertrophy at injection site was common with impure animal insulin. They are rarely seen with purified human insulin. Allergic rash at injection-site or hematoma are uncommon with human insulin. Infection at site of insulin pump has been described.

Stretching of skin as a result of fluid accumulation is seen over legs in patients who are on TZD (Glitazones).

## SKIN INFECTIONS IN DIABETIC PATIENTS

- Bacterial-cellulites, furunculosis on the nape of the neck
- Foot infection–superficial or deep
- Paronychia

Fungal
- Vulvovaginitis or balanitis
- Tinea paedis
- Erosive interdigitalis

## SKIN LESIONS HAVING HIGHER INCIDENCE IN DIABETICS

Vitiligo is found to be more common in diabetics. There is total loss of melanin from some areas of the skin leading to chalky white appearance. Lesions are patchy and are well demarcated. They are bi-laterally symmetrical. They could be near natural orifices. Flexor areas are more involved as opposed to extensor areas.

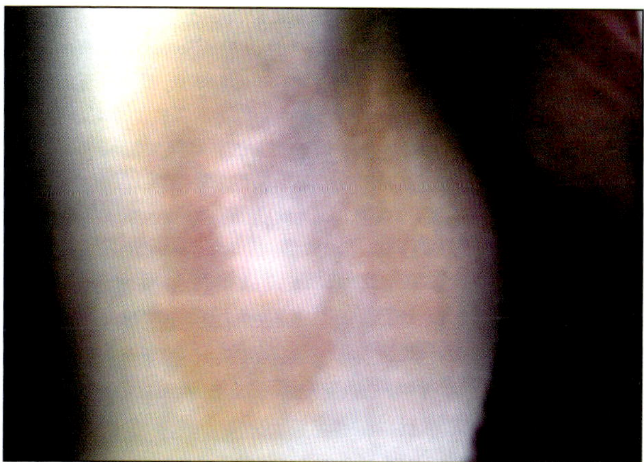

**Figure 27.1:** Acanthosis in armpit

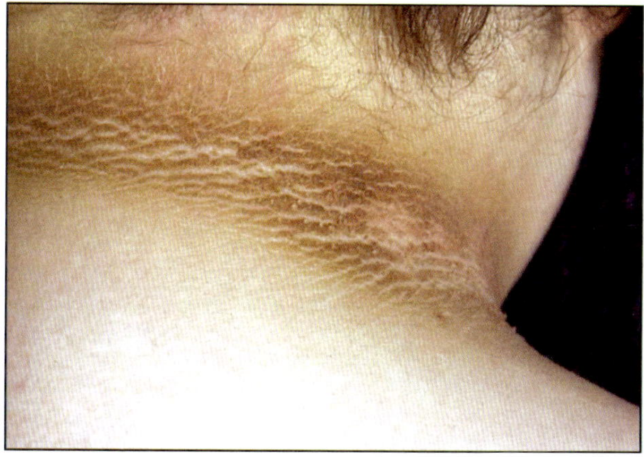

**Figure 27.2:** Acanthosis on nape of the neck

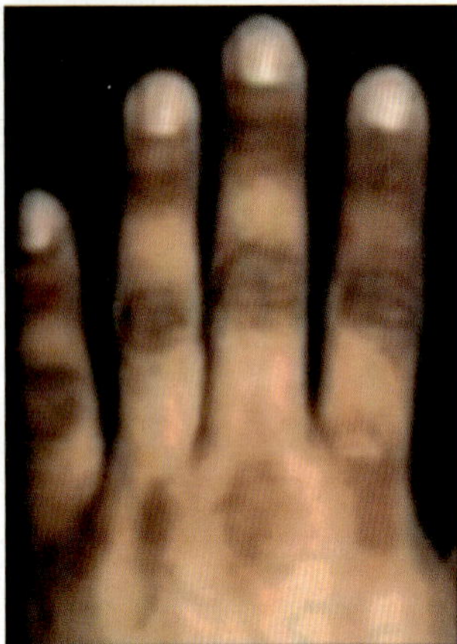

**Figure 27.3:** Acanthosis on knuckles

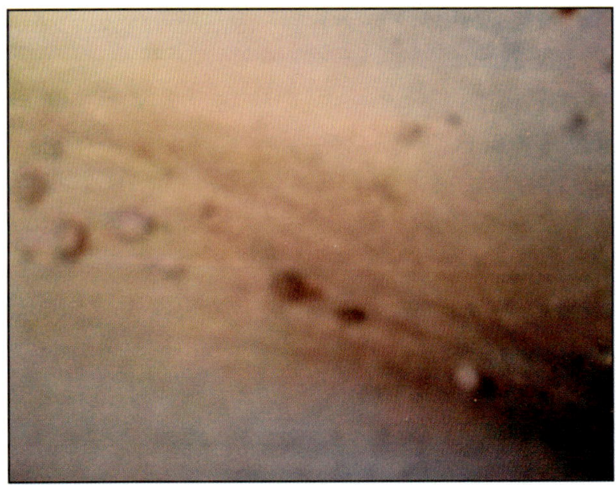

**Figure 27.4:** Skin tags in acanthosis

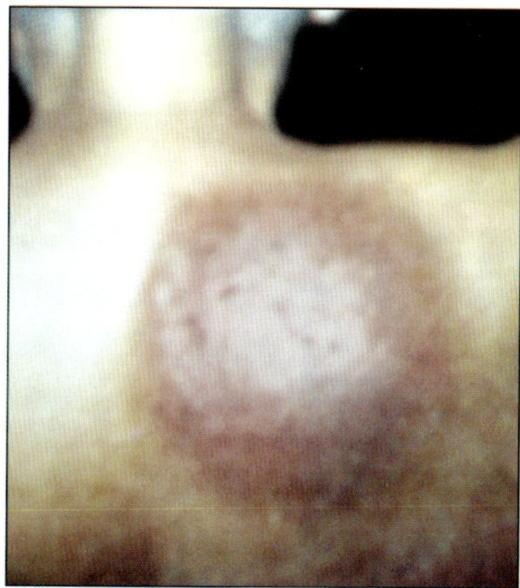

**Figure 27.5:** Carbuncle on back

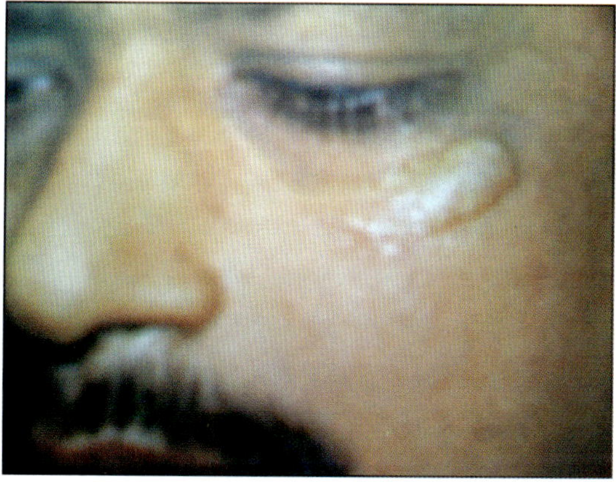

**Figure 27.6:** Xanthelasma

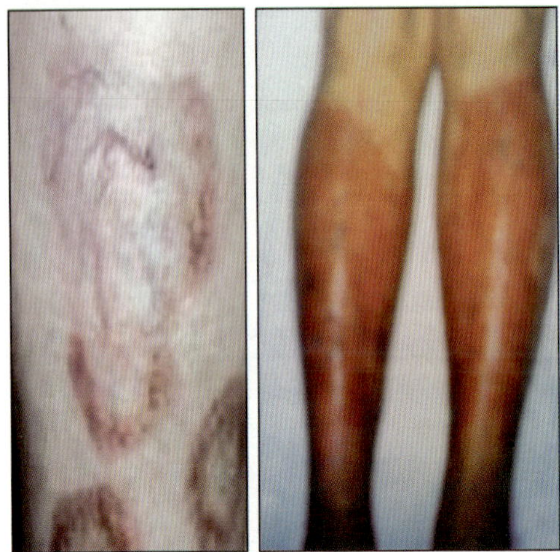

**Figure 27.7:** Necrobiosis lipoidica diabeticorum (NLD)

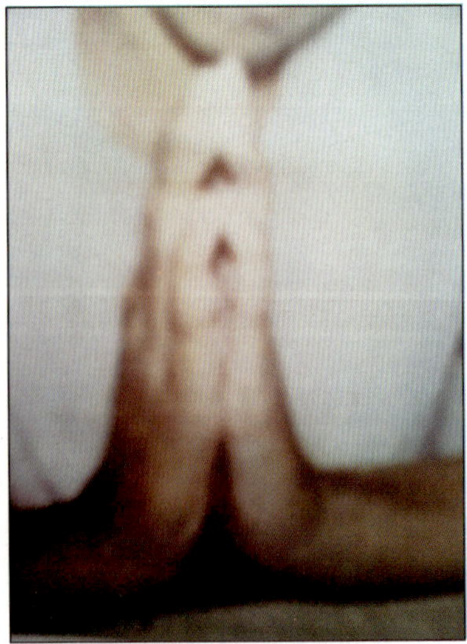

**Figure 27.8:** Namaste sign

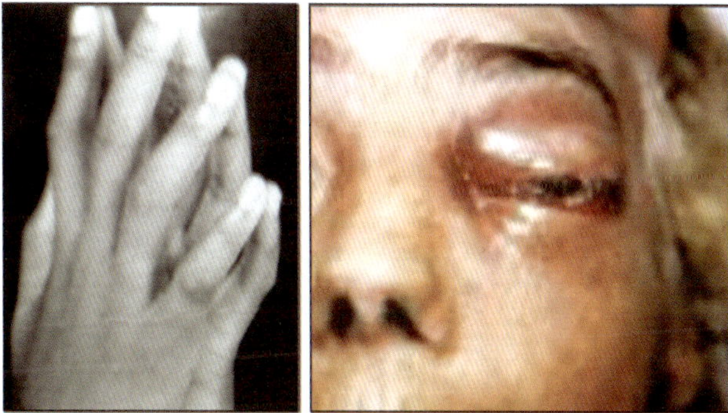

**Figure 27.9:** Prayer sign, Mucormycosis

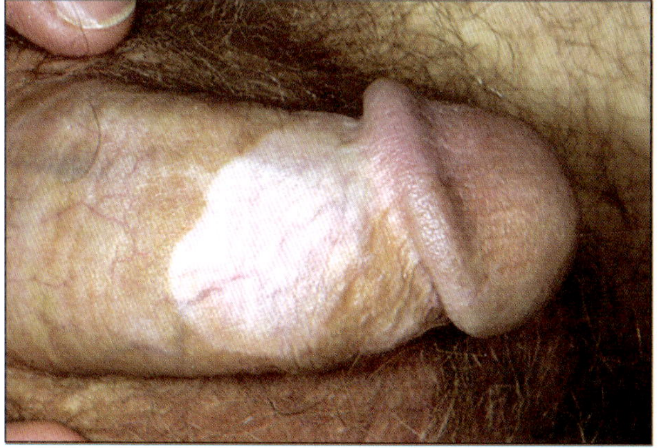

**Figure 27.10:** Penile vitiligo

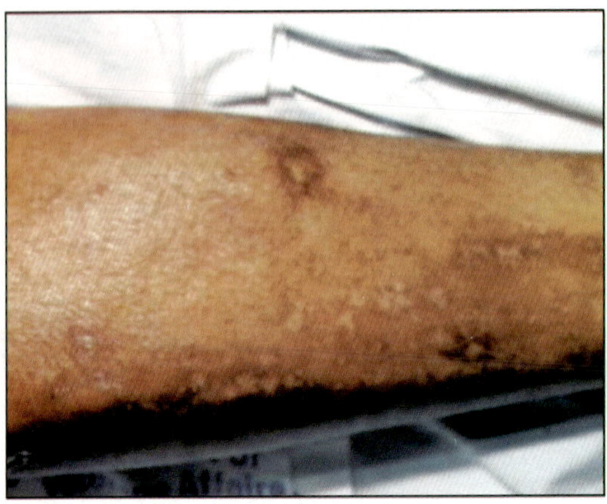

**Figure 27.11:** Diabetic dermopathy

Skin lesions found in diabetic patient are of wide variety. Alert physician will be able to diagnose them in most of the cases. Many of them do not have very effective therapy. But adequate reassurance after correct diagnosis is usually sufficient for the patient.

# Chapter 28

# Hypoglycemia

Correct diagnosis of Hypoglycemia is possible by using Whipple's triad. It includes:

- Symptoms and signs suggestive of Hypoglycemia
- Low plasma blood glucose that corresponds to symptoms
- Resolution of symptoms with correction of plasma glucose.

Usual cut of point to diagnose hypoglycemia is 70 mg/dl (approx. 3.9 mMol). Some people use 55 mg/dl (3 mMol) as a cut off. DCCT and UKPDS have shown that tight blood sugar control reduces microvascular complications but the risk of hypoglycemia goes up. Surgical patients are benefited by tight glycemic control during ICU and hospital stay but similar results were not seen in medical ICU cases. The NICE-Sugar study has shown that very tight glycemic control increases the risk of hypoglycemia and its morbidity and mortality.

## SYMPTOMS

- Sympatho-Adrenergic occur at early phase of hypo-tremors, sweating, nausea, hunger, anxiety, palpitations and tachycardia.
- Neuroglucopenic – usually appear late, confusion, dizziness, altered sensorium, visual disturbances, altered speech, inability to concentrate, amnesia, delirium in some cases, mood changes, semiconsciousness, hemiparesis, convulsions, coma, death.

## CLINICAL SETTINGS

- Excessive dose of medication- intentional or unknowingly especially common with insulin and sulfonylurea (SU) drugs
- Too much of exercise–Over enthusiasm to control hyperglycemia rapidly
- Less food intake or acute gastroenteritis
- Alcohol overdose
- Organ failure–hepatic or renal
- During septicemia
- Addison's disease, insulinoma
- Nesiodoblastosis after bariatric surgery
- After gastric bypass or result of gastroparesis due to DAN
- Autoimmune–antibodies to insulin or to insulin receptors.

## DIAGNOSIS

It is confirmed by measuring plasma or whole blood sugar level. Blood sugar less than 70 mg% is diagnostic when it is associated with symptoms. Urine sugar is of no use to diagnose hypoglycemia.

Fasting hypoglycemia could be because of insulinoma. It is diagnosed by measuring insulin levels, C-peptide levels, pro-insulin to insulin ratio, glucagon stimulation test and imaging techniques like MRI or endoscopic ultrasound.

## TREATMENT

Rapid administration of simple sugars either orally or by Intravenous drip.

In resistant hypoglycemia subcutaneous glucagon is useful.

Alpha-glucosidase inhibitors (AGI) slow down the process of breaking down of complex sugars to simple sugars. Patients on these agents should be instructed to consume dextrose (Glucon-D) and not cane sugar during hypoglycemia.

## HYPOGLYCEMIA PREVENTION

One single episode of hypo-reduces the perception level for next hypoglycemic episode. Person may get recurrent sub clinical episodes of hypoglycemia resulting into minor cerebral insults. Hence, prevention of hypoglycemia is very important.

Proper education about diabetes, frequent self monitoring of glucose, flexible schedule of hypoglycemic agents targeting individual glucose goals along with constant professional support will prevent hypoglycemia in vast majority of cases.

Dose of insulin or SU drugs should be correctly chosen and patient should be instructed about making minor alteration in dosage depending upon his diet-pattern and exercise level. Instructions about precise timing of food intake should be given considering the pharmacokinetics of medications administered. In most of the situations 20-30 minutes gap should be observed between insulin and SU dose. Person on AGI should take food immediately after taking the tablet. Titration of rapid or intermediate acting insulin dosage should be done depending upon timing of hypoglycemia.

Excessive exercise should be discouraged. Slow and steady upgradation helps to achieve smooth control.

OHA or insulin should be stopped or taken in smaller dose during short periods of illness when food intake has drastically reduced. Person having vomiting and diarrhea should be watchful about symptoms of hypoglycemia.

Person taking alcohol in moderate to heavy amount should be instructed to consume sufficient food in order to avoid late hypoglycemia.

All diabetics should carry an ID which contains their personal information like name address and emergency contact number. It should also contain instructions in simple regional language in case the person carrying this ID is found semiconscious or comatose. Simple measures like this will ensure timely treatment during hypoglycemia.

**Front Side of Diabetes ID (HYPO-ID)**
**DIABETES IDENTITY CARD**

Name: ——————————————
Address:——————————————
——————————————
——————————————
——————————————

Emergency contact number: ——————————————
Contact number of family physician ——————————————
Contact number of diabetes consultant: ——————————————

**Rear Side of Diabetes ID (HYPO-ID)**
**Please read this card to save my life!**

I am a diabetic person.

In case I am found to have profuse sweating, trembling or if you feel that my behavior is abnormal or if you find me in semiconscious state, then kindly give me sugar to eat or drink immediately.

Emergency contact numbers are printed on the rear side of this card. Please inform my family members and doctors immediately.

Chapter 29

# Drug-induced Hyperglycemia and Hypoglycemia

Diabetic person needs various medicinal agents other than oral hypoglycemic agents for the comorbid conditions. Although majority of these agents are prescribed by medical professionals, use of over the counter medications and unscientific or traditional remedies cannot be ignored when one thinks of drug induced hyperglycemia or hypoglycemia. Some endocrine conditions do disturb glucose equilibrium. People with metabolic syndrome do have insulin resistance and more prone to develop hyperglycemia.

Information hereafter is provided in tabular form

| *Drug category and note* | *Mechanism of action and special features* |
|---|---|
| • Anti-psychotics<br>Olanzapine, clozapine<br>chlorpromazine, haloperidol<br>sertraline, tricyclic agents | More common with newer drugs<br>– Augment IR, suppress beta cells<br>– Less frequent<br>– Very rare |
| • Anti-hypertensive agents<br>Diuretics – Thiazide<br>– Loop diuretics<br>– Spironolactone<br>Beta blockers – Propranolol<br>– Metoprolol, atenolol<br>– Carvedilol<br><br>Calcium channel blockers | Many diabetics need these agents<br>Hypokalemia → insulinopenia<br>Mechanism unknown<br>Does not cause hyperglycemia<br>Cause insulinopenia<br>Less common<br>Improves insulin sensitivity →<br>Improves glucose control<br>Causes insulinopenia |
| • Anti-inflammatory agents<br>Glucocorticoids (Topical creams can raise glucose)<br>indomethacin, glucosamine | <br>Increase hepatic glucose output and increase insulin resistance<br>Mechanism not known |
| • Sympathomimetics and neuromodulatory agents<br>– Terbutaline injection<br>– Poisoning with rogor<br>– Organophosphorous | Glycogenolysis and gluconeogenesis<br>Augment IR, suppress beta cells<br>When used in premature labor<br>Irreversible beta cell destruction |

*Contd...*

*Contd...*

| *Drug category and note* | *Mechanism of action and special features* |
|---|---|
| – Endosulfan | – At times hypoglycemia<br>By central nervous system stimulation |
| • Immunomodulatory agents<br>Cyclosporine, tacrolimus. Especially when used with steroids<br>Protease Inhibitors, didanosin, stavudine | Used during organ transplant<br>Beta cell dysfunction and augment IR<br><br>Augment IR, induce adiposity<br>Attack beta cells, hypokalemia |
| • Antibiotics<br>– Gatifloxacin<br>– Pentamidine | Infection augments IR<br>Variable effect on glucose<br>Injury to beta cells |
| Alcohol | Chronic ingestion of more than 3 drinks per day, augments IR |
| Nicotine, caffeine, catecholamine | Augment IR, suppress beta cells |
| Nicotinic acid | Increase gluconeogenesis |
| Cimetidine, phenytoin | Reduce insulin secretion |
| Quinine | Glycogenolysis |
| Morphine | Increases glucagon secretion |
| Overdose of aspirin, paracetamol, isoniazide, theophyline | Reversible condition |
| TPN | Underlying insulin resistant state |
| Growth hormone (GH) | Insulin like activity |
| Testosterone | Augment IR |
| Estrogen | Increase GH and cortisol |
| Progesterone | Reduce number and affinity of insulin receptors |
| Catecholamines | Antagonize insulin action, augment glucagon secretion |

Patients use various traditional medicines regularly. Information about such usage is often not disclosed to the treating physician. One has to ask about these agents specifically when desired stable glucose control is not achieved. Many of such agents do contain heavy metals like lead. Some impairment in renal function is likely to occur with these agents. A patient will start experiencing hypoglycemia with concomitant use of traditional medicines. He feels happy but soon he lands up in renal failure. Physician has to remain alert about this possibility as various promotional materials readily available on television or internet lure or misguide our diabetics.

Chapter 30

# Metabolic Emergencies in Diabetes

Diabetic person can face critical metabolic derangements, which could be either hyperglycemic or hypoglycemic. Hypoglycemia has been discussed separately in chapter of this book. Hyperglycemic emergencies include diabetic ketoacidosis and hyperosmolar nonketotic coma (HONK) or hyperglycemic hyperosmolar syndrome (HHS). Lactic acidosis though rare deserves special mention.

## DIABETIC KETOACIDOSIS (DKA)

It is more common in type I diabetics but type II diabetics are not totally immune. The commonest cause of DKA is missing a dose of insulin. Pump failure is upcoming cause with more and more pump usage. Other causes include infection, acute myocardial infarction, very intense and prolonged exercise, pancreatitis, trauma, surgery, heavy dosage of steroids or antipsychotics, stroke, acute thrombosis or bleeding, and cocaine use.

Both type I and type II diabetics can manifest with DKA as a presenting feature.

Absolute insulin deficiency leads to hyperglycemia and hyperlipemia. Former gives rise to osmotic symptoms and the later one leads to ketoacidosis.

Clinical features include those of severe hyperglycemia (polyuria, polydipsia) followed by abdominal pain, vomiting, labored breathing, dehydration and semi-consciousness. If not detected early then the outcome is poor. At times DKA is mistaken for acute abdominal emergencies by surgeons.

Laboratory results reveal high blood sugar > 350 mg%, ketonuria, low blood pH, low bicarbonates, high potassium (initial phase) near normal sodium, low chlorides. Anion gap (Measured sodium level minus total of chloride and bicarbonate - Na – (Cl + $HCO_3$) more than 12 is seen. Tests for ketones in blood (Beta-Hydroxy butyric acid- B-OHB) are rccommended as a specific test for DKA but it is not available in most of the centers. WBC count is raised. ECG should be done to rule out silent myocardial infarction. Slight elevation of blood urea and creatinine level is noted. Chest X- ray and blood/urine culture studies should be done if clinically indicated.

Differential diagnosis includes methanol poisoning, starvation ketosis, alcoholic ketoacidosis, and septicemia.

Treatment includes rapid re-hydration and insulinization. Normal saline should be infused very rapidly 1-1.5 lit in first 30 minutes ideally guided by CVP line. It is followed by half liter of normal saline in 2 hours and subsequently more gradual replacement of fluid should be carried out.

Insulin should be administered via a separate intravenous line, if possible with the help of infusion pump. Serum potassium level should be above 3.3 mEq/l before initiating insulin supplementation. Initial bolus of 10-20 units of rapid action insulin may be given intravenously. Main part of therapy is intravenous insulin drip or infusion 10 units per hour (0.14 U/kg). Blood sugar should be measured every one hourly. Insulin is continued till the blood sugar drops below 200 mg% and there is reduction in ketonuria. It is followed by glucose – insulin potassium drip to correct hypokalemia. Potassium supplementation is not needed if serum potassium is above 5.3 mEq/L.

Appropriate antibiotics should be given to tackle infection. Intravenous soda-bicarb is given only in severe cases with very low bicarbonate levels (less than 5 mEq/L). Phosphate replacement is not recommended as a routine.

Flow chart to note clinical parameters and glycemic state is very useful for modifying treatment plans. As the clinical condition improves, patient can be shifted to subcutaneous insulin.

### Key Points in Treatment of DKA

- Rapid fluid replacement
- Intravenous insulin
- Monitor potassium
- Treat underlying cause
- Sodabicarb replacement.

Indicators of bad prognosis are unconsciousness, blood pH below 7.1, persistent acidotic breathing and hypotension. Overall prognosis is good in majority of cases with DKA if detected early and managed aggressively.

### Bad Prognostic Signs in DKA

- Unconsciousness
- Acidotic breathing
- pH below 7.1
- Hypotension

Complications of DKA are hypoglycemia, hypokalemia, cerebral edema, rhabdomyolysis, thromboembolism, and pulmonary edema.

## HONK (HHS)

This complication is more common in elderly people who have limited access to health care. Severe dehydration is the hallmark of this condition. Altered mental state dominates clinical picture. Relative insulin deficiency is noted. Absent or minimal ketosis is seen. Blood sugars are very high in the range of 800-1200 mg%. Water deficit is about 9 liter as opposed to 6 liter in DKA. Arterial pH is usually 7.3; Bicarb levels are above 15 mEq/L. Anion gap is less than 12. Serum osomlality (2 × measured sodium plus glucose level divided by 18), i.e. 2 × (Na + glucose)/18. is above 320 Osm/kg.

Fluid deficit in HONK is more severe but caution should be exercised in replacing fluids rapidly in older patients who have limited cardiac and renal reserve. Insulin is needed in intravenous form and is continued till plasma glucose is 250 mg/l, osmolality is below 320 and improvement in mental state is seen.

Prognosis of HONK (HHS) is not as good as that of DKA that carries less than 1% mortality. The reasons for higher mortality in HONK include age, delay in initiating therapy and associated comorbid conditions.

## LACTIC ACIDOSIS

Lactic acidosis is a serious but fortunately rare complication of metformin therapy in type II diabetes. It was more common with phenformin use, the drug that is no longer available. It is especially common when metformin is used inappropriately in patients with renal or cardiac dysfunction. It leads to hypotension and cardiac failure. Mortality of lactic acidosis is 50%, but fortunately the incidence of lactic acidosis is 0.03 per 1000 patient-years of treatment.

Chapter 31

# Screening Schedule for Comorbidities of Diabetes

## HYPERTENSION

- Check blood pressure at every visit. Normal range is below 130 (Systolic), 80 (Diastolic). Recheck on next day if reading is high.
- Check blood pressure in sitting, lyingdown and standing position in patients with neuropathy.
- Rule out white coat hypertension
- Use 24 hrs ambulatory blood pressure monitoring in selected cases.

## DYSLIPIDEMIA

Measure fasting lipid profile at diagnosis and then once a year.

14 hrs fasting is desirable.

*Target:* Cholesterol < 200 mg /dl, LDL < 70 mg/dl for high-risk cases and < 100 for low-risk cases. HDL > 50 mg/dl and triglycerides < 150 mg %.

## CHD RISK

- Evaluate various cardiometabolic risk factors for CHD once a year.
- Pay special attention to nicotine use, lack of physical activity, central obesity apart from hypertension, microalbuminuria and dyslipidemia.
- Baseline ECG is advisable in all cases.
- 2 D echo, Treadmill test, coronary angiography or perfusion scan when clinically indicated.

## NEPHROPATHY SCREENING

Once a year testing urine for albuminuria is desirable, preferably for microalbuminuria.

Serum creatinine estimation and calculation of glomerular filtration rat (GFR) once a year. Calculate albumin-creatinine ratio.

## RETINOPATHY SCREENING

Comprehensive eye check-up, once a year for all diabetics above 10 years of age.

More frequent follow-up is needed in those with progressive retinal disease.

Diabetic woman with pregnancy should have full eye check-up during 1st trimester and subsequently during pregnancy and one year postpartum.

## NEUROPATHY SCREENING

- Clinical tests for neuropathy at diagnosis and every year thereafter.
- Electrophysiological tests are rarely needed.
- Screen for autonomic neuropathy at diagnosis and then every 5 years.

## FOOT CARE

- Annual comprehensive foot examination to identify foot at risk.
- Use 128 Hz tuning fork, monofilament, hot and cold water in test tubes and test for VPT by biosthesiometer.
- Look for peripheral pulses.
- Enquire about nicotine and alcohol use.

## HYPOTHYROIDISM

Screen patients with type I diabetes for thyroid peroxidase and thyroglobulin antibodies at diagnosis.

Measure TSH in type II diabetics once in 2-3 years.

# Chapter 32

# Surgery in Diabetes

Diabetic person may need surgical interventions in his life. The surgery could be for the peculiar conditions peculiar to the disease like foot gangrene or it could be one of those performed in non-diabetic subjects, e.g. cataract removal, renal transplant, CABG or appendicectomy. Nearly half of the diabetic population needs surgical assistance for their health problems and nearly one-fifth of them face some complication during perioperative period.

Perioperative complications in diabetic patient

| *Infections* | *Bacterial* |
|---|---|
| Metabolic | Like hyper or hypoglycemia, hypo or hyperkalemia, ketosis |
| Cardiovascular | Like hypotension, arrhythmia, myocardia infarction, CHF |
| Renal | Like acute renal shutdown or volume overload |

Pathophysiological factors, which play important role during perioperative period in a diabetic person, are high level of counter-regulatory hormones like glucagon, cortical, catecholamines and growth hormone leading increased hepatic glucose output, increased lipolysis, depressed peripheral uptake of glucose leading to high levels of blood glucose and free fatty acids.

Duration and extent of tissue handling, stress of surgery, prolonged fasting state lead to altered glucose metabolism.

A surgeon before taking up the case for surgery, asks preoperative evaluation. For medicolegal reasons it is better to note down risk category of the patient rather than declaring the patient as fit or unfit for anesthesia. The surgeon, anesthetist, the patient and the relatives should take the final decision about surgery jointly.

## PREOPERATIVE EVALUATION

Preoperative evaluation should include:

- Detailed history especially duration of diabetes, habit of tobacco/alcohol, degree of overall control, cardiac symptoms, symptoms of peripheral neuropathy, etc.
- Assessment of metabolic control by latest blood sugar levels, HbA1C report, S. electrolytes, nutritional status of the person.
- Cardiovascular assessment is done by measuring blood pressure in lying down position, in standing and in sitting positions, to rule out postural hypotension, baseline ECG and 2D echo in high-risk cases. Treadmill testing for cardiac function is needed in very selected cases.
- Neurological assessment is vital because impaired gastric motility increases the risk of aspiration and may delay the absorption of enteral feeds during post-operative period. Postural hypotension and poor emptying of bladder can pose problems too.
- Renal function should be assessed prior to surgery by relevant blood and urine tests. Abnormal renal function should caution the physician about chances of fluid overload, changes in potassium levels in diabetic person who is on insulin-glucose drip.

## ROLE OF INSULIN IN PERIOPERATIVE PERIOD

- Preoperative period to normalize blood glucose level quickly and smoothly.
- Intraoperative period to minimize fluctuations in glucose levels.

- Postoperative period to maintain blood glucose levels below acceptable level without causing hypoglycemia.

All patients with type I diabetes, insulin requiring type II diabetics and those who need general anesthesia for surgery should receive glucose—insulin infusion during perioperative period. Insulin can be administers with 5 or 10% glucose solution or can be given separately by syringe pump. When you are giving insulin in glucose solution, one should prepare 3 different bags of varying insulin concentration ranging from 10 to 30 units. Frequent blood sugar monitoring by glucometer will guide the selection of proper drip for that moment. At times glucose and insulin can be administered through single vein but from two different bags. This offers more flexibility. Subcutaneous insulin, if any, must be discontinued in these patients.

## INSULIN GLUCOSE PROTOCOL

| *Blood glucose in mg/dl* | *Insulin infusion units per hour* | *5% Dextrose ml/hour* |
|---|---|---|
| < 70 | 0.5 | 150 |
| 71-100 | 1.0 | 125 |
| 101-150 | 2.0 | 100 |
| 151-200 | 3.0 | 50 |
| 201-250 | 4.0 | Nil |
| 251-300 | 6.0 | Nil |
| Above 300 | 10.0 | Nil |

- Very high doses of insulin are needed in patients undergoing cardiac surgery.
- Potassium supplementation should be given along with insulin-glucose infusion.

- 10% dextrose is preferred over dextrose 5% in those patients, who are at risk of fluid overload.
- Target for blood glucose for immediate postoperative period is 100-125 mg/dl and later on it should be maintained below 180 mg/dl.

## MANAGEMENT OF BLOOD SUGAR WHEN ORAL INTAKE IS ALLOWED

Stop insulin infusion half an hour after giving subcutaneous insulin.

Measure blood glucose fasting, before every meal, at bedtime and at 3 AM.

Use short acting insulin in doses appropriate for blood sugar.

| *Blood glucose in mg/dl* | *Insulin dose at breakfast* | *Insulin dose at lunch* | *Insulin dose at dinner* | *Insulin dose at bedtime* |
|---|---|---|---|---|
| <71 | 03 | 02 | 02 | 00 |
| 71-100 | 04 | 03 | 03 | 00 |
| 100-150 | 06 | 04 | 04 | 00 |
| 151-200 | 08 | 06 | 06 | 00 |
| 201-250 | 10 | 08 | 08 | 01 |
| 251-300 | 12 | 10 | 10 | 02 |
| Above 301 | 14 | 12 | 12 | 03 |

Person on total parenteral nutrition may need insulin infusion for a day or so. Later on total daily dose of insulin can be added to infusion bag. These people need insulin in very high dose (100U per day).

Other facets of postoperative care include:

- Attention to electrolyte balance
- Cardiac assessment especially in older patients.
- Early ambulation or antithrombotic measures
- Intake output charts
- Wound care
- Avoiding pressure sores
- Chest physiotherapy.

Proper attention to glucose control, electrolytes, fluid management, cardiac status and would hygiene will give very good postoperative results in a person with diabetes.

Chapter 33

# Prevention of Diabetes

Diabetes is spreading like a wild fire in developing countries. India is going to be capital of diabetes by the year 2025. People from our country with low earning per head and hence they will find it very difficult to manage complications of diabetes. If we start doing some serious thinking about prevention strategies for noncommunicable diseases like diabetes, ischemic heart disease, then the epidemic of these medical problems will be arrested or slowed down to some extent.

Prevention of diabetes is considered in three sub-headings:

- Primary prevention will reduce prevalence of diabetes
- Secondary prevention will reduce morbidity out of diabetes
- Tertiary prevention will reduce death due to complications of diabetes.

## PRIMARY PREVENTION

Primary prevention is possible if our society members follow the 10 commandments listed below:

- Food intake should match the physical activity of the person.
- Raw food should form sizeable portion of diet.
- Control intake of oil, butter, ghee (Margarine), salt and sugar, jaggery, honey.
- Pulses, green leafy vegetables and select fresh fruits should be consumed routinely.
- Avoid foods that contain preservatives. Avoid processed food as far as possible.

- Daily exercise for 20 minutes should be fitted in everybody's timetable, no matter how busy the person is.
- Nicotine causes insulin resistance. Stay away from nicotine in any form. Avoid caffein before 9 AM.
- Know the limitations of social drinking. If you have successfully stayed away from alcohol then do not start alcohol (not even wine) for so called "health benefits".
- Learn to manage stress. It will reduce sympathetic outflow.
- Avoid marriages between two families with strong family history of diabetes.

Pharmacological agents are used in various clinical trials conducted for diabetes prevention. It is debatable whether you are really preventing the problem, delaying it or using pharmacological agents for the condition that is yet to appear. Majority of studies were carried out in people with Impaired Glucose Tolerance (IGT).

Agents that are found to be useful are:

- Metformin—Diabetes Prevention Program
- Ramipril—HOPE trial
- Rosiglitazone—DREAM trial
- Acarbose—STOP-NIDDM trial
- Orlistat—XENDOS study.

## SECONDARY PREVENTION

Secondary prevention includes prevent, delay or slow down complications of diabetes. The complications microvascular like neuropathy, retinopathy or nephropathy or macrovascular like ischemic heart disease, cerebrovascular disease or peripheral vascular disease or a mixed one like diabetic foot gangrene or few typical clinical conditions which are particularly seen in diabetics like periarthritis shoulder, rhinocerebral mucormycosis.

Majority of these conditions are prevented by tight glucose control along with control of blood pressure, regulating lipid levels and staying away from nicotine. Proper education of the patient and family members is very important in this matter. It will ensure regular check-ups, compliance or adherence to medication, regularity in exercise, total de-addiction and proper diet. All these combined will result in steady metabolic state, which will benefit the diabetic person and his family in long run.

Monitoring of diabetes should go much beyond blood sugar estimation. Lipid profile, creatinine, S GPT (S ALT), microalbuminuria, complete blood count, complete urine examination (Discourage urine sugar testing), ECG, comprehensive eye check-up should be carried out at diagnosis and must be repeated every year in asymptomatic cases. The frequency of repeating the abnormal test should be more, especially in symptomatic patient. Good clinical history and thorough clinical examination should be carried out as routine at follow-up visits. Things like proper measurement of blood pressure, looking for early signs of neuropathy or congestive heart failure require special attention. All these will enable early detection of major complications.

Addition of specific agents at early stage of disease will prevent future downhill journey. ACE inhibitors and Angiotensin Receptor Blockers (ARB) are known to reduce proteinuria and to have nephroprotective effect. Aspirin and lipid lowering agents have shown to reduce cardiovascular morbidity. B-complex preparations do not have sufficient data to prove their role in reversing or slowing down neuropathy. Sildenafil will benefit a diabetic male to correct erectile dysfunction. It will help in boosting his confidence and restoring disturbed marital life. Early detection of diabetic retinopathy, ideally in nonproliferative stage, will allow a clinician some time to preserve remaining retina by photocoagulation. Early detection of glucose abnormality during pregnancy will prevent fetal loss or macrosomia. Proper care of innocent looking foot ulcer will preserve the foot.

## TERTIARY PREVENTION

Tertiary prevention is focused on preventing death due to complications of diabetes. Cardiovascular disease is responsible for half of the deaths in diabetic population while end stage renal disease is responsible for nearly 1/3rd of deaths. Timely revascularization, aggressive medical management, renal replacement therapy will prevent such situation. A diabetic person will thus be able to enjoy life to its fullest length, with some limitations of course.

## DO TELL YOUR PATIENT FOLLOWING LINES?

- Having diabetes can be considered as an accident.
- Taking proper care of diabetes is responsibility.
- Neglecting it purposefully is unpardonable crime which will definitely be punished by the Almighty.

## COMMUNITY-BASED PREVENTIVE STRATEGIES

- Selecting people at risk – relatives of a diabetic person, overweight, those having sedentary lifestyle and those who use nicotine.
- Promoting concept of healthy eating right from school days.
- Explaining importance of physical activity.
- Simple means to increase physical activity in daily routine like using staircase instead of an elevator, walking during lunch-break or while reaching the office, etc.
- Teach them to say NO to nicotine.

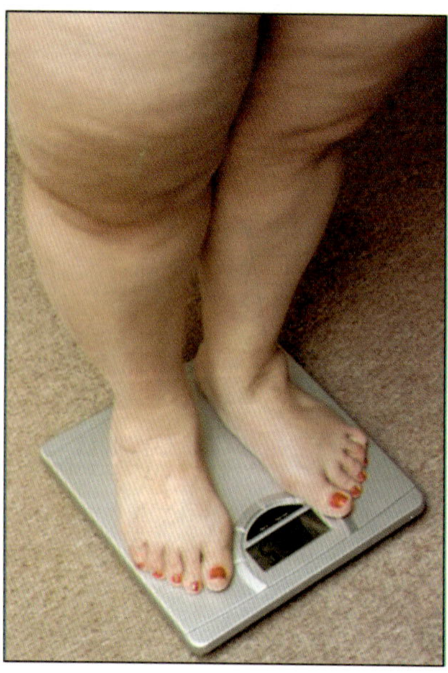

**Figure 33.1**

Combining efforts of policymakers. Government-machinery, social organizations, spiritual leaders or movie actors/actresses (as they have tremendous mass appeal), teachers and of those actively involved in providing health care will definitely give us victory in war against diabetes.

Chapter 34

# Gestational Diabetes Mellitus

Gestational diabetes mellitus, (GDM) is a condition in which women without previously diagnosed diabetes exhibit high blood glucose levels for the first time during pregnancy.

Gestational diabetes generally has few symptoms and it is most commonly diagnosed by screening during pregnancy. Gestational diabetes affects 3-10% of pregnancies, depending on the population studied. No specific cause has been identified, but it is believed that the hormones produced during pregnancy increase a woman's resistance to insulin, resulting in impaired glucose tolerance. There is some role of genetic predisposition too. Insulin resistance is superimposed upon by beta cell dysfunction leading to high blood glucose.

Babies born to mothers with gestational diabetes are at increased risk of problems typically such as being large for gestational age (which may lead to delivery complications), neonatal hypoglycemia and jaundice. Gestational diabetes is a treatable condition and women who have adequate control of glucose levels can effectively decrease these risks.

Women with gestational diabetes are at increased risk of developing type II diabetes mellitus after pregnancy, while their offspring are prone to developing childhood obesity, with type 2 diabetes later in life. Most patients are treated only with diet modification and moderate exercise but some need insulin.

## DEFINITION

Gestational diabetes is formally defined as any degree of glucose intolerance with onset or first recognition during pregnancy. This definition acknowledges the possibility that patients may have previously undiagnosed diabetes mellitus, or may have developed diabetes coincidentally with pregnancy. Whether symptoms subside after pregnancy is also irrelevant to the diagnosis.

## EPIDEMIOLOGY

The frequency of gestational diabetes varies widely by study depending on the population studied. It occurs in between 5 and 10% of all pregnancies (between 1-14% in various studies).

## PATHOPHYSIOLOGY

The precise mechanisms underlying gestational diabetes remain unknown. The hallmark of GDM is increased insulin resistance. Pregnancy hormones and other factors are thought to interfere with the action of insulin as it binds to the insulin receptor. Additional amount of insulin is needed to overcome this resistance; about 1.5-2.5 times more insulin is produced in a normal pregnancy.

Insulin resistance is a normal phenomenon emerging in the second trimester of pregnancy, which progresses thereafter to levels seen in non-pregnant patients with type 2 diabetes. It is thought to secure glucose supply to the growing fetus. Women with GDM have an insulin resistance and they cannot compensate with increased production in the beta cells of the pancreas. Placental hormones, and to a lesser extent increased fat deposits during pregnancy, seem to mediate insulin resistance during pregnancy. Cortisol and progesterone are the main culprits, but human placental lactogen, prolactin and estradiol contribute too.

It is unclear why some patients are unable to balance insulin needs and develop GDM, however a number of explanations have been given, similar to those in type 2 diabetes: Autoimmunity, single gene mutations, obesity, and other mechanisms.

Because glucose travels across the placenta (through diffusion facilitated by GLUT3 carriers), the fetus is exposed to higher glucose levels. This leads to increased fetal levels of insulin. The growth-stimulating effects of insulin can lead to excessive growth and a large body (macrosomia). After birth, the high glucose environment disappears, leaving these newborns with ongoing high insulin production and susceptibility to hypoglycemia.

## RISK FACTORS AND SYMPTOMS

Classical risk factors for developing gestational diabetes are the following:

- Previous diagnosis of gestational diabetes or pre-diabetes, impaired glucose tolerance, or fasting hyperglycemia.
- Family history of type 2 diabetes.
- Maternal age—over 35 years.
- Ethnic background (those with higher risk factors include African-Americans, Afro-Caribbean, Native Americans, Hispanics, Pacific Islanders, and people originating from the Indian subcontinent).
- Overweight, obese or severely obese.
- Previous pregnancy which resulted in a child with a high birth weight (> 90th percentile, or >4000 g (8 lbs 12.8 oz))
- Poor obstetric history
  - Smoking, PCOD.
  - Short stature.

About 40-60% of women with GDM have no demonstrable risk factor; for this reason many advocate to screen all women. Typically women with gestational diabetes exhibit no symptoms (another reason for universal screening), but some women may have complaints like increased thirst, increased urination, fatigue, nausea and vomiting, urinary tract infection and blurred vision.

## SCREENING AND DIAGNOSIS

A number of screening and diagnostic tests have been used to look for high levels of glucose in plasma or serum in defined circumstances. One method is a stepwise approach where a suspicious result on a screening test is followed by diagnostic test. Alternatively, a more involved diagnostic test can be used directly at the first antenatal visit in high-risk patients (for example in those with polycystic ovarian syndrome or Acanthosis nigricans).

### Tests for Gestational Diabetes

- Non-challenge blood glucose tests
- Screening glucose challenge test
- Oral glucose tolerance test (OGTT).

Non-challenge blood glucose tests involve measuring glucose levels in blood samples without challenging the subject with glucose solutions. A blood glucose levels is determined when fasting, 2 hours after a meal, or simply at any random time. In contrast challenge tests involve drinking a glucose solution and measuring glucose concentration thereafter in the blood; in diabetes they tend to remain high. The glucose solution has a very sweet taste that some women find unpleasant; sometimes therefore artificial flavors are added. Some women may experience nausea during the test, and more so with higher glucose levels.

### Screening Pathways

There are different opinions about optimal screening and diagnostic measures, in part due to differences in population risks, cost-effectiveness considerations, and lack of an evidence base to support large national screening programs. The most elaborate regime entails a random blood glucose test during a booking visit, a screening glucose challenge test around 26 weeks gestation, followed by an OGTT if the tests are outside normal limits. If there is a high suspicion, women may be tested earlier.

In the United States, most obstetricians prefer universal screening with a screening glucose tolerance test. In the United Kingdom, obstetric units often rely on risk factors and a random blood glucose test. The American Diabetes Association and the Society of Obstetricians and Gynecologists of Canada recommend routine screening unless the patient is low risk (this means the woman must be younger than 25 years and have a body mass index less than 27, with no personal, ethnic or family risk factors).

### Non-challenge Blood Glucose Tests

When a plasma glucose level is found to be higher than 126 mg/dl (7.0 mMol/l) after fasting, or over 200 mg/dl (11.1 mMol/l) on any occasion, and if this is confirmed on a subsequent day, the diagnosis of GDM is made, and no further testing is required. These tests are typically performed at the first antenatal visit. They are patient-friendly and inexpensive, but have a lower test performance compared to the other tests, with moderate sensitivity, low specificity and high false positive rates.

### Screening Glucose Challenge Test

The screening glucose challenge test (sometimes called the O'Sullivan test) is performed between 24-28 weeks, and can be seen as a simplified version of the oral glucose tolerance test (OGTT). It involves drinking a solution containing 50 grams of glucose, and measuring blood levels 1 hour later.

If the cut-off point is set at 140 mg/dl (7.8 mMol/l), 80% of women with GDM will be detected. If this threshold for further testing is lowered to 130 mg/dl, 90% of GDM cases will be detected, but there will also be more women who will be subjected to a consequent OGTT unnecessarily.

### Oral Glucose Tolerance Test (OGTT)

OGTT should be done in the morning after an overnight fast of between 8 and 14 hours. During the three previous days the subject must have an unrestricted diet (containing at least 150 g carbohydrate per day) and unlimited physical activity. The subject should remain seated during the test and should not smoke throughout the test.

The test involves drinking a solution containing a certain amount of glucose, and drawing blood to measure glucose levels at the start and on set time intervals thereafter.

The diagnostic criteria from the National Diabetes Data Group (NDDG) have been used most often, but some centers rely on the Carpenter and Coustan criteria, which set the cutoff for normal at lower values. Compared with the NDDG criteria, the Carpenter and Coustan criteria lead to a diagnosis of gestational diabetes in 54% more pregnant women, with an increased cost and no compelling evidence of improved perinatal outcomes.

The following are the values, which the American Diabetes Association considers to be abnormal during the 100 g of glucose OGTT:

- Fasting blood glucose level ≥ 95 mg/dl (5.33 mMol/l)
- 1 hour blood glucose level ≥ 180 mg/dl (10 mMol/l)
- 2 hours blood glucose level ≥ 155 mg/dl (8.6 mMol/l)
- 3 hours blood glucose level ≥ 140 mg/dl (7.8 mMol/l)

### *Complications*

GDM poses a risk to mother and child. This risk is largely related to high blood glucose levels and its consequences. The risk increases with higher blood glucose levels. Treatment resulting in better control of these levels can reduce some of the risks of GDM considerably.

The two main risks GDM imposes on the baby are growth abnormalities and chemical imbalances after birth, which may require admission to a neonatal intensive care unit. Infants born to mothers with GDM are at risk of being both large for gestational age (macrosomia) and small for gestational age. Macrosomia in turn increases the risk of instrumental deliveries (e.g. forceps and cesarean section) or problems during vaginal delivery (such as shoulder dystocia). Macrosomia may affect 12% of normal women compared to 20% of patients with GDM. However, the evidence for each of these complications is not equally strong; in the hyperglycemia and adverse pregnancy outcome (HAPO) study for example, there was an increased risk for babies to be large but not small for gestational age. Research into complications for GDM is difficult because of the many confounding factors (such as obesity). Labeling a woman as having GDM may but not necessarily increase the risk of having a cesarean section.

Neonates are also at an increased risk of hypoglycemia, jaundice, polycythemia, hypocalcemia and hypomagnesemia. GDM also interferes with maturation, causing dysmature babies prone to respiratory distress syndrome due to incomplete lung maturation and impaired surfactant synthesis.

Unlike pregestational diabetes, gestational diabetes has not been clearly shown to be an independent risk factor for birth defects. Birth defects usually originate sometime during the first trimester (before the 13th week) of pregnancy, whereas GDM gradually develops and is least pronounced during the first trimester. Studies have shown that the offspring of women with GDM are at a higher risk for congenital malformations. A large case control study found that gestational diabetes was linked with a limited group of birth defects, and that this association was generally limited to women with a higher body mass index ($\geq 25\ kg/m^2$). It is difficult to make sure that this is not partially due to the inclusion of women with pre-existent type 2 diabetes who were not diagnosed before pregnancy.

Because of conflicting studies, it is unclear at the moment whether women with GDM have a higher risk of pre-eclampsia. In the HAPO study, the risk of pre-eclampsia was between 13% and 37% higher, although not all possible confounding factors were corrected.

Prognosis gestational diabetes generally resolves once the baby is born. Based on different studies, the chances of developing GDM in a second pregnancy are between 30 and 84%, depending on ethnic background. A second pregnancy within 1 year of the previous pregnancy has a high rate of recurrence.

Women diagnosed with gestational diabetes have an increased risk of developing diabetes mellitus in the future. The risk is highest in women who needed insulin treatment had GAD or islet cell antibodies, women with more than two previous pregnancies, and women who were obese (in order of importance). Women requiring insulin to manage gestational diabetes have a 50% risk of developing diabetes within the next five years. Depending on the population studied, the diagnostic criteria and the length of follow-up, the risk can vary enormously. The risk appears to be highest in the first 5 years, reaching a plateau thereafter.

Children of women with GDM have an increased risk for childhood and adult obesity and an increased risk of glucose intolerance and type 2 diabetes later in life. This risk relates to increased maternal glucose values. It is currently unclear how much genetic susceptibility and environmental factors each contribute to this risk, and if treatment of GDM can influence this outcome.

## Classification

The White classification is widely used to assess maternal and fetal risk. It distinguishes between gestational diabetes (type A) and diabetes that existed prior to pregnancy (pregestational diabetes). These two groups are further subdivided according to their associated risks and management.

There are 2 subtypes of gestational diabetes (diabetes which began during pregnancy):

- Type A1: Abnormal oral glucose tolerance test (OGTT) but normal blood glucose levels during fasting and 2 hours after meals; diet modification is sufficient to control glucose levels.
- Type A2: Abnormal OGTT compounded by abnormal glucose levels during fasting and/or after meals; additional therapy with insulin or other medications is required.

### Treatment

The goal of treatment is to reduce the risks of GDM for mother and child. Scientific evidence is beginning to show that controlling glucose levels can result in less serious fetal complications (such as macrosomia) and increased maternal quality of life. Unfortunately, treatment of GDM is also accompanied by more infants admitted to neonatal wards and more inductions of labor, with no proven decrease in cesarean section rates or perinatal mortality.

Counseling before pregnancy (for example, about preventive folic acid supplements) and multidisciplinary management are important for good pregnancy outcomes. Most women can manage their GDM with dietary changes and exercise. Self-monitoring of blood glucose levels can guide therapy. Some women will need insulin therapy.

Any diet needs to provide sufficient calories for pregnancy, typically 2,000-2,500 kcal with the exclusion of simple carbohydrates. The main goal of dietary modifications is to avoid peaks in blood sugar levels. This can be done by spreading carbohydrate intake over meals and snacks throughout the day, and using slow-release carbohydrate sources known as the GI diet. Since insulin resistance is highest in mornings, breakfast carbohydrates need to be restricted more.

Regular moderately intense physical exercise is advised, although there is no consensus on the specific structure of exercise programs for GDM.

Target ranges are as follows:

- Fasting capillary blood glucose levels < 5.5 mMol/l ≈ 100 mg/dl.
- 1 hour postprandial capillary blood glucose levels <8.0 mMol/l ≈ 144 mg/dl.
- 2 hours postprandial blood glucose levels <6.7 mMol/l ≈ 120 mg/dl. (1 mMol = 18.0 mg of glucose).

Regular blood samples can be used to determine HbA1C levels, which give an idea of glucose control over a longer time period.

If monitoring reveals failing control of glucose levels with these measures, or if there is evidence of complications like excessive fetal growth, treatment with insulin might become necessary. The most common therapeutic regime involves premeal fast-acting insulin to blunt sharp glucose rises after meals. Care needs to be taken to avoid hypoglycemia due to excessive insulin injections. Insulin therapy can be normal or intensive; more injections can result in better control but requires more effort, and there is no consensus that it has large benefits.

There is some evidence that certain oral glycemic agents might be safe in pregnancy, or at least, are significantly less dangerous to the developing fetus than poorly controlled diabetes. However, few studies have been performed as of this time and this is not a generally accepted treatment. These agents may be used in research settings, or if the patient needs intervention but refuses insulin therapy, and is aware of the risks. Glyburide, second generation sulfonylurea, has been shown to be an effective alternative to insulin therapy. In one study, 4% of women needed supplemental insulin to reach blood sugar targets.

Metformin has shown promising results. Treatment of polycystic ovarian syndrome with Metformin during pregnancy has been noted to decrease GDM levels. A recent randomized controlled trial of Metformin versus insulin showed that women preferred Metformin tablets to insulin injections, and that Metformin is safe and equally effective as insulin. Severe neonatal hypoglycemia was less common in insulin-treated women, but preterm delivery was more common. Almost half of patients did not reach sufficient control with Metformin alone and needed supplemental therapy with insulin; compared to those treated with insulin alone, they required less insulin, and they gained less weight. There remains a possibility of long-term complications from Metformin therapy, although follow-up at the age of 18 months of children born to women with polycystic ovarian syndrome and treated with Metformin revealed no developmental abnormalities.

If a diabetic diet or GI diet, exercise, and oral medication are inadequate to control glucose levels, insulin therapy may become necessary.

The development of macrosomia can be evaluated during pregnancy by using sonography. Women who use insulin, with a history of stillbirth, or with hypertension are managed like women with overt diabetes.

Research suggests a possible benefit of breastfeeding to reduce the risk of diabetes and related risks for both mother and child.

A repeat OGTT should be carried out 2-4 months after delivery, to confirm the diabetes has disappeared. Afterwards, regular screening for type 2 diabetes is advised.

Chapter 35

# Insulin Injection Techniques

The very thought of injecting yourself with insulin takes a little getting used to, and doing it properly requires some practice. But once the patient has taken the first dose, then insulin injection will quickly become a regular part of the daily routine.

Injecting at the proper depth is an important part of good injection technique. Most health care professionals recommend that insulin be injected in the subcutaneous fat. If one injects too deep, the insulin could go into muscle, where it is absorbed faster but might not last so long (and, it hurts more when you inject into muscle). If the injection is not deep enough, the insulin goes into the skin, which affects the insulin's onset and duration of action.

Most people pinch up a fold of skin and insert the needle at a 60°-90° angle to the skin fold. To pinch your skin properly, follow these steps:

- Squeeze a couple of inches of skin between your thumb and two fingers, pulling the skin and fat away from the underlying muscle (If you use a 5 millimeters mini-pen needle to inject, you do not have to pinch up the skin when injecting at a 90° angle; with this shorter needle, you do not have to worry about injecting into muscle.)
- Insert the needle.
- Hold the pinch so the needle does not go into the muscle.
- Push the plunger (or button if you are using a pen) to inject the insulin.
- Release the grip on the skin fold.
- Remove the needle from the skin.

Note that not everyone injects at a 90° angle. If you inject into an area of the body that has less fat, you may need to inject at less than a 45° angle, to avoid injecting into a muscle.

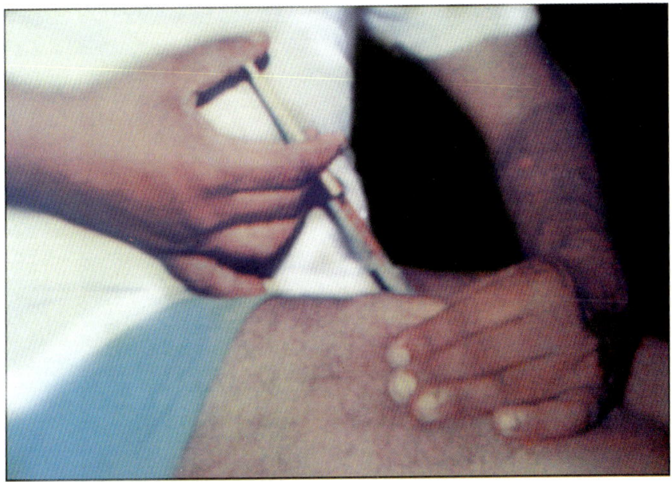

**Figure 35.1:** Most preferred site-outer side of thigh

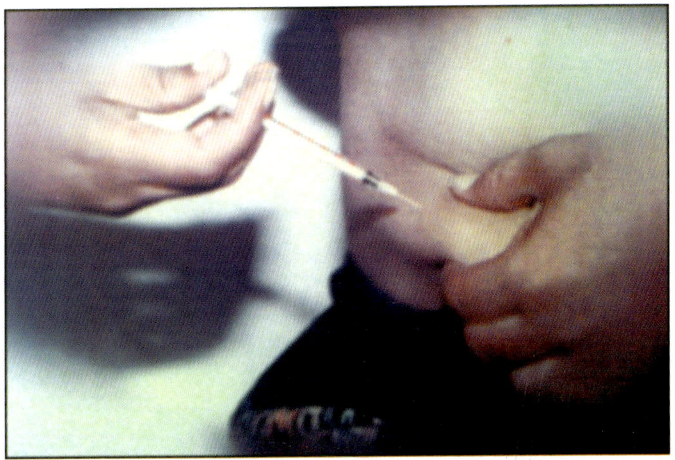

**Figure 35.2:** Next choice on abdomen

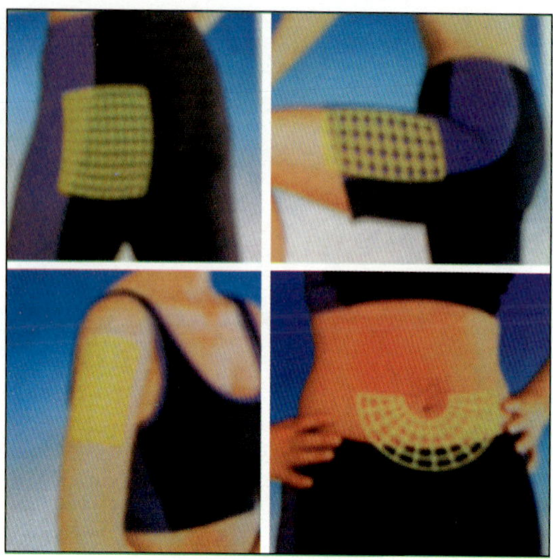

**Figure 35.3:** Other sites

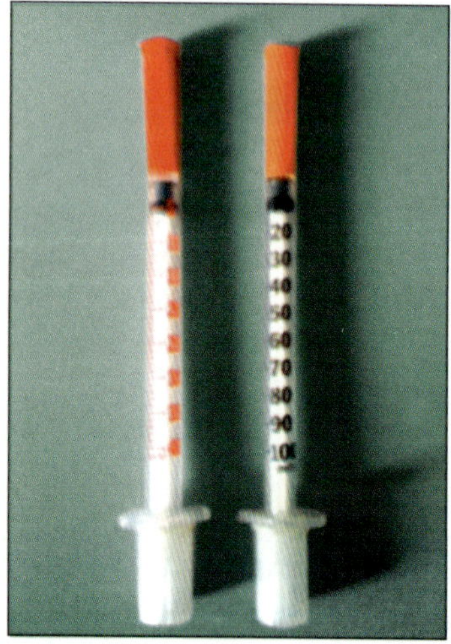

**Figure 35.4:** Syringes–U40 and U100

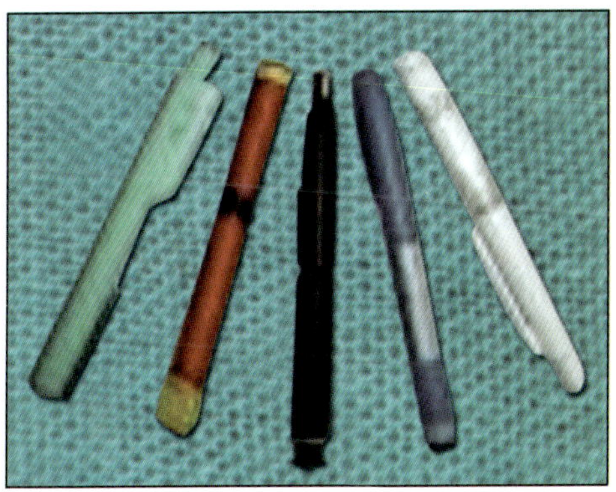

**Figure 35.5:** Insulin pens

The angle you should use to insert the syringe or pen needle into your body depends on your body type, the injection site, and the length of the needle that you use.

# Appendices

# APPENDIX I

## DRUGS CAUSING HYPERGLYCEMIA

- Psychiatric agents
  Olanzapine, clozapine
  Chlorpromazine, haloperidol
  Sertraline, tricyclic agents
- Anti-hypertensive agents
  Diuretics – thiazide and loop diuretics
  Beta blockers – propranolol, Metoprolol, Atenolol
- Anti-inflammatory agents
  Glucocorticoids even topical creams can raise glucose
  indomethacin, glucosamine
- Sympathomimetics and neuromodulatory agents
- Poisoning with rogor
  - Organophosphorous
  - Endosulfan
- Immunomodulatory agents
  Cyclosporine, tacrolimus, especially when used with steroids
  Protease inhibitors,
  Didanosin, stavudine
- Antibiotics
  - Gatifloxacin (Variable effect)
  - Pentamidine
- Others
  Alcohol—chronic use
  Nicotine, caffeine, catecholamine
  Nicotinic acid
  Cimetidine, phenytoin
  Quinine
  Morphine

Overdose of aspirin, paracetamol, isoniazide, theophyline
TPN
Growth hormone (GH)
Testosterone
Estrogen
Progesterone
Catecholamin

# APPENDIX II

## EMPIRICAL ANTIBIOTICS FOR INFECTIONS IN DIABETES

| *System involved* | *Organism* | *Initial treatment* | *Advanced treatment* |
|---|---|---|---|
| **1. Urinary Tract** | | | |
| Acute cystitis or urethritis | *E. Coli*, *S.Saphrophyticus* | Fluroquinolones | TMP + SMZ |
| | *Enterococci* | Ampicillin | Vacomycin |
| Acute pyelonephritis | *E. Coli* | Fluroquinolones<br>Ceftazideine, ampicillin | Ticarcillin+<br>Clavulanate<br>Piperacillin+<br>Tazobactum |
| Perinephric abscess | E.Coli | As above | As above |
| S.aureus bacteremia | S.aureus | Nafcillin/oxacillin | Cefazolin vacomycin |
| **2. Foot infection** | | | |
| Acute non-limb threatening | *S.aureus*, streptococci | Clindamycin<br>Cephalosporin<br>Ampicillin + Clavulanate | ———— |
| Chronic | Polymicrobial<br>*S.aureus*, streptococci,<br>*E.coli, Proteus,*<br>*Klebsiella*<br>Anaerobes | Ampicillin + Sulbactum<br>Ticarcillin + Clavulanate<br>Piperacillin + Tazobactum<br>Clindamycin + Cefotaxime | |
| Limb threatening | As above | Imipenem + Cilastatin<br>Meropenem + Vacomycin | |
| Narcotizing fascitis | Group B strepto.<br>Clostridia | Penicillin G + Clindamycin<br>Imipenem + Cilastatin<br>Meropenem | |
| **3.Abdomen** | | | |
| Cholecystitis | Enterococci,<br>bacteroids | Piperacillin + Tazobactum<br>Ampicillin + Sulbactum<br>Ticarcillin + Clavulanate | |

# APPENDIX III

## CARDIAC PERFUSION STUDIES

### Single-photon Emission Computed Tomography

*Myocardial Perfusion Imaging in Patients with Diabetes*

Diabetes mellitus has reached epidemic proportions, creating a large population of people at increased risk for cardiac events. Single-photon emission computed tomography myocardial perfusion imaging (SPECT MPI) provides an effective tool to accurately diagnose and risk stratify patients with diabetes, similar to patients without diabetes. Diabetics, however, are at increased risk for coronary events. Diabetics with normal MPI have increased late cardiac events, and even those with mild perfusion defects have increased event rates compared with non-diabetics with similar perfusion abnormalities.

Stress MPI can provide valuable risk stratification data for both the sexes, with or without diabetes. However, diabetes appears to exert a greater relative impact in women than in men. Despite the absence of symptoms, the incidence and prevalence of coronary artery disease is increased in patients with diabetes.

Myocardial perfusion single-photon emission computed tomography (MP-SPECT) has become essential for screening diabetic patients at high risk of silent myocardial ischemia. The combined use of pharmacological and exercise stress, together with the generalization of gated studies has increased both the sensitivity and the specificity of MP-SPECT, leading to a better identification of balanced coronary artery disease, of coronary artery disease with normal coronary angiography, and artifacts. In addition, the incremental prognostic value of gated MP-SPECT over myocardial perfusion and clinical data has been demonstrated.

## RECENT IMPROVEMENTS IN MP-SPECT

Although myocardial perfusion imaging has been available in routine clinical settings since the 1970s, the development of gated SPECT over the past two decades has made a possible combined assessment of myocardial perfusion and left ventricular function.

This additional information on ventricular function has proven to be useful for both the diagnosis and prognosis of CAD. Using gated studies, the quantification of post-stress wall motion abnormalities or ejection fraction increases the sensitivity of stress-rest.

MP-SPECT, especially in patients with three vessel CAD, in whom a diffuse decrease in sub-endocardial blood flow may cause an impairment of ventricular function without focal perfusion defects. Moreover, quantification of wall motion is a powerful tool which helps us to differentiate actual scars from attenuation artifacts, thus leading to better specificity of gated MP-SPECT compared with non gated studies.

Finally, post-stress left ventricular ejection fractions and end-systolic volumes measured by gated MP-SPECT are independent predictors of cardiovascular events and have incremental prognostic values over myocardial perfusion and clinical data in predicting cardiac death.

These recent advances in MP-SPECT have been enhanced by improvements in the stress procedure used, especially for patients with diabetes, who are less likely to achieve peak stress using conventional procedures than are non- diabetic patients. It has been shown that the combined use of a vasodilator-induced pharmacological stress (intravenous dipyridamole or adenosine) and sub-maximal exercise on a treadmill or bicycle reduces the non cardiac side effects of vasodilatation and arrhythmias while producing images that are similar to that produced when maximal exercise is achieved.

### Which diabetic patients should be screened for silent myocardial ischemia?

Diabetic patients have a high incidence of occult CAD, ranging from 20% to nearly 60%, depending on the patient populations included in the various study groups. The risk of cardiac death, myocardial infarction, or revascularization is more than 7-fold greater in diabetic patients with myocardial perfusion defects than in diabetic patients with normal scintigraphic data.

The European and American guidelines recommend screening asymptomatic diabetic patients with evidence of peripheral or carotid occlusive arterial disease, microvascular disease (proliferative retinopathy, nephropathy), or at least two cardiovascular risk factors (diabetic dyslipidemia, hypertension, smoking, family history of premature CAD.

Although the emerging evidence supports the appropriateness of testing patients with vascular disease recent studies have reported a similar frequency of abnormal MP-SPECT studies in asymptomatic diabetic patients with and without two or more cardiovascular risk factors.

## THALLIUM OR SESTAMIBI STRESS TESTS

Alternative Names-Sestamibi and thallium stress tests.

### MIBI Stress Test

Thallium and sestamibi stress tests are nuclear imaging methods that provide a view of the blood flow into the heart muscle, both at rest and during activity.

These tests are also called MIBI stress test and myocardial perfusion scintigraphy.

### How the Test is performed?

This test is done at a nuclear medicine center. You will be told to exercise according to your effort tolerance on a treadmill or bicycle.

After reaching your maximum level of exercise, the doctor will inject a radioactive material into a vein, usually either thallium or sestamibi. The material will travel in the bloodstream, through the coronary arteries, and into the heart muscle in accordance with the coronary flow at that time as you complete your exercise session. Once inside the heart muscle, the radiotracer does not come out of it.

Next, you will lie down on a table under a special camera that scans the heart and detects the radioactive material. A computer will look at how the material has collected and create pictures of the heart. The first pictures are made shortly after the exercise test, which shows blood flow to the heart during exercise. This part is called a "stress test"

You will be again given the same tracer when you are at rest and again more pictures of your heart are taken. These images show blood flow through your heart during rest.

If your doctor does not think exercise is safe for you, or if you have joint problems that may make doing so difficult, you will be given a drug called a vasodilator that will make your heart feel as if you were exercising. This medicine widens normal blood vessels to the heart, which increases blood flow. Arteries with blockages remain narrow, and therefore will receive less blood. After you receive this medicine, you will receive the radioactive material, as described above. The test done using a vasodilator can potentially show a heart problem in the same way as the exercise test.

### Why the Test is performed?

The thallium and sestamibi stress tests are indicated when your doctor needs to evaluate, for example:

- How does your heart responds to exercise?
- The cause of your chest pain.
- The degree of blockage in your coronary arteries
- What to expect after you have had a heart attack
- How well a heart procedure done to improve blood flow in your coronary arteries is working

### Normal Results

When a normal amount of the radiotracer arrives into all areas of the heart, then the images obtained are normal. The heart images at peak exercise are compared to the heart images at rest. If during both exercise and rest all images are normal, then your blood flow through the coronary arteries is considered to be normal.

### What does an abnormal results mean?

In your heart pictures, an area may lack the radiotracer and thus show a spot of a different color, called a "defect". Defects represent poor uptake of the radiotracer by the heart because of reduced blood flow. When a defect occurs at peak exercise and not at rest, the most likely cause is a significant blockage of a coronary artery. When a defect is observed both at rest and with exertion, then it indicates that previous damage from a heart attack has occurred and that the heart muscle has a scar. In case the defect is reversible, you will be advised to go for angioplasty or bypass depending upon the number of vessels showing defects.

### Risks

Nuclear imaging stress tests are very safe. Radiation exposure to radiotracers can be a concern for the nuclear lab staff, but not for patients undergoing an occasional nuclear imaging test.

# APPENDIX IV

Please note: 1 katori = 25 grams raw daal/rice = 1 small bowl
1 chapatti = 25 grams flour

## STANDARD DIET CHARTS FOR DIABETICS

### 1800 Kcal Diet Chart

- *Early morning:* Tea/coffee – 1 Cup [without sugar and milk without cream] + 2 Marie Biscuits
- *Breakfast:* Poha/Upma – 1 plate [without groundnut and coconut] OR Paratha (60 grams flour) [stuffed with vegetables] made on non-stick pan – 1 no. + 1 Katori curd
  OR Dosa chutney – 2 medium size
  [chutney without groundnut and coconut]
  OR Idli Sambar – 3 medium size + 1½ Katori Sambar
  OR Daliya Upma – 1½ Katori
  OR Chapatti + Vegetable – 2 + 1½ Katori vegetable
  + 1 Cup milk [without sugar and milk without cream]
- *Mid morning:* Fruit [Apple, Sweet lime, Orange, Guava, Watermelon, Pomegranate, Papaya {2-3 pieces}, Jambhul {7-8}, Fig {wet}]
- *Lunch:* Salad – 1 Katori [Cucumber, Carrot, Radish, Onion, Tomato]
  {With curd (75 grams) and without groundnut and coconut}
  + Chapatti – 2 no. (60 grams flour)/Phulka – 4 no./Bhakri – 1 no. [Jowar, Nagli]
  + Vegetable – 1 ½ Katori
  + Rice – ½ Katori
  + Daal/Usal – 1 katori (25 grams raw)
  + Curd – 1 katori/buttermilk – 1 katori

- *Afternoon snacks:* Tea/Coffee – 1 Cup [without sugar and milk without cream] + 2-3 Marie biscuits + 1 fruit
  OR Rice flakes/Puffed rice chiwda – 1½ katori
  [Without groundnut, coconut, shev, farsan]
  OR Jowar flakes – 1½ K
  OR Rajgira flakes – 1½ K
  OR Sprout bhel – 1 K [with Cucumber, Onion, Tomato, Sprouts should be steamed]
  OR Brown bread vegetable sandwich – 2 slices
  [Once in a week]
- *Dinner:* Same as lunch but chapatti should be eaten in less quantity and rice should be avoided in dinner.
- *Bedtime:* 1 Cup milk [without sugar and milk without cream]
- *Energy:* 1848 Kcal, Proteins – 73.2 gm, CHO – 286 gm, Fats – 41 gm

[Note – when nonvegetarian food is consumed avoid daal and Usal, i.e. pulses].

# APPENDIX V

Please note: 1 katori = 25 grams raw daal/rice
1 chapatti = 25 grams flour

## 1600 KCAL DIET CHART FOR DIABETIC

- *Early morning:* Tea/Coffee – 1 cup [without sugar and milk without cream] + 2 Marie biscuits
- *Breakfast:* Poha/Upma – 1 plate (50 grams) [without groundnut and coconut]
  OR Thalipith – 1 medium size (60 grams) with curd – ½ Katori (75 grams)
  OR Tomato omlette – 2 [Medium size and made of mix flours]
  OR Paratha flour) (50 gms [stuffed with vegetables] made on nonstick pan – 1 no.
  + ½ Katori curd
  OR Chapatti + Vegetable –1½ no. + 1 Katori
  + 1 Cup milk [without sugar and milk without cream]
- *Mid morning:* Fruit [Apple, Sweet lime, Orange, Guava, Watermelon, Pomegranate, Papaya {2-3 pieces}, Jambhul {7-8}, Fig {wet}
- *Lunch:* Salad – 1 Katori [Cucumber, Carrot, Radish, Onion, Tomato] + Chapatti – 2 (50 grams flour)/Phulka – 3 no./Bhakri – ¾ [Jowar, Nagli]
  + Leafy vegetable – 1½ K or Other vegetable – 1 K
  + Daal/Usal – 1 Katori (25 grams raw) [with less oil about ½ tsp.]
  + Rice –(50 grams raw) ½ K
- *Afternoon snacks:* Tea/Coffee – 1 Cup [without sugar and milk without cream] + 2 Marie biscuits + 1 Fruit
  OR Khakara – 2 no. {without oil}
  OR Rice Flakes/Puffed Rice Chiwda – 1½ Katori

[Without groundnut, coconut, shev, and farsan]
OR Jowar flakes – 1½ K
OR Sprout Bhel – ½ K
[With cucumber, onion, tomato, sprouts should be steamed]

- *Dinner:* Same as lunch but chapatti should be eaten in less quantity and rice should be avoided in dinner.
- *Bedtime:* 1 cup milk [without sugar and milk without cream]
- *Energy:* 1549 Kcal, Proteins–56 gm, CHO – 221 gm, Fats–35 gm

[Note – when nonvegetarian is consumed avoid daal and Usal, i.e. pulses].

# APPENDIX VI

Please note: 1 katori = 25 grams raw daal/rice
1 chapatti = 25 grams flour

## 1200 KCAL DIET CHART FOR DIABETIC

- *Early morning:* Tea/Coffee – 1 Cup [without Sugar and Milk without Cream]
- *Breakfast:* Poha/Upma – 1 Katori [without Groundnut and Coconut]
  OR Steamed sprouts – 1 Katori [with Cucumber, Onion, Tomato]
  OR Phulka + Vegetable – 2 no. + 1 Katori
  OR Egg white – 2
  OR Idli Sambar – 2 medium size + 1 Katori Sambar
  + 1 Cup skim milk
- *Mid Morning:* Fruit [Apple, Sweet lime, Orange, Guava, Watermelon, Pomegranate, Papaya {2-3 pieces}, Jambhul {7-8}, Fresh Fig
- *Lunch:* Salad – 1 Plate [Cucumber, Carrot, Radish, Onion, Tomato]
  + Buttermilk – 1 Glass [thin]
  + Phulka –(30 grams flour) 2 no.
  OR Bhakri – ½
  + Leafy Vegetable – 1½ K or Other vegetable – 1 K
  + Daal/Usal – 1 K [daal plain]
  + Rice – ½ K [twice or thrice a week only]
- *Afternoon snacks:* Tea/Coffee – 1 Cup [without sugar and milk without cream]+ 2 Marie biscuits + 1 fruit
  OR Khakara – 1 no. {without oil}
  OR Rice flakes/Puffed Rice Chiwda – 1 Katori
  [Without groundnut, coconut, shev, and farsan]
  OR Jowar flakes – 1 K

- *Dinner:* Same as lunch but chapatti should be eaten in less quantity and rice should be avoided in dinner.
- *Bedtime:* 1-Cup skim milk
- *Energy:* 1220 Kcal, Proteins – 53 gm, CHO – 170 gm, Fats – 23 gm

[Note – when nonvegetarian is consumed avoid daal and usals, i.e.pulses]

# APPENDIX VII

## SOME INTERESTING RECIPES FOR DIABETICS

### NUTRITIOUS KHEER

#### Ingredients

- Sprouted wheat – 1 katori/bowl
- Sprouted nagli – 1 katori
- Barley – 1 katori
- Milk – 1 katori

#### Method

- Dry the sprouted wheat and nagli for 4 days in shade.
- Mix barely in the above mixture and make flour of it.
- Take 1 katori milk, 1 katori water and 1 tbsp. above flour mix well and bring it to boil.
- After it is boiled remove from fire, add sugar free substitute and serve.

### DIABETIC CARAMEL CUSTARD

#### Ingredients

- 2-½ cup low fat milk
- 1 tbsp. custard powder
- 3 sachets sugar free substitute
- ½ tbsp. vanilla essence
- 5 gm china grass [agar agar], cut into small pieces.
- 1 tbsp. sugar for caramelizing.

### Low Fat Milk

Boil the milk and skim the fat layer [malai] that is formed after it has been cooled repeat this procedure for at least twice to get fat free milk.

### Method

- Soak the china grass in ¾ cup of cold water for 15-20 mins. Put to cook on slow flame until it dissolves. Keep warm.
- In a pudding mould, add the sugar [for caramelizing] and 1 tbsp. of water and continue cooking until the sugar becomes brown. Spread the caramelized sugar all over the base of the mould, rotating the mould to spread in evenly. The sugar will harden quickly.
- Mix the custard powder in ½ cup of cold milk.
- Boil the remaining milk. When it comes to boil, add the custard powder and milk mixture and continue cooking till you get a smooth sauce.
- Add the china grass solution to the custard and boil again for 2 minutes.
- Strain the mixture and cool it slightly [Strain the mixture if it is lumpy].
- Add the vanilla essence and sugar substitute and mix well. Pour this mixture over prepared pudding mould. Allow it to set in refrigerator.
- Before serving, loosen the sides with a sharp knife and invert on a plate. Serve chilled.

## SPROUTED MOONG PULAO

### Ingredients

- Unpolished rice—1 cup
- Sprouted moong—1½ cup

- Onion chopped—1 no.
- Green chilies—1 finely chopped
- Spinach [finely chopped]—1½ cup
- Oil -1 tbsp.
- Cinnamon—2 sticks
- Bay leaf—2 no.
- Cumin seeds—½ tbsp.
- Cloves—2 no.
- Salt to taste.

### Method

*For the rice*—heat the oil and fry the bay leaves, cumin seeds, cinnamon and cloves for few minutes. Add washed rice, salt and fry for 2-3 minutes. A tea cup of water, cover and cook.

*For the sprouts*—heat oil and fry the onion and green chilies for 2 minutes. Add sprouts and cook for 2-3 minutes. Add the spinach and cook again for a min. add the cooked rice and mix well. Serve hot.

## OATS TIKKI

### Ingredients

- Instant oats – 1 cup
- Sprouted moong – 1 cup
- Chopped Spinach – 1 cup
- Boiled potato – 1 no.
- Green chilies paste – 1 tbsp.
- Goda masala – 1 tbsp.
- Ginger garlic paste – 1 tbsp.
- Coriander powder and Jeera powder – 1 tbsp.
- Dry mango powder – 1 tbsp.
- Oil – 2 tbsp.

- Coriander leaves
- Salt to taste.

### Method

- Steam chopped spinach and sprouts, do not over cook.
- Add little oil in frying pan to fry oats. Grind the sprouted moong in mixer and make a rough paste.
- Smash potato, add moong paste, steamed spinach, ginger garlic and green chilies paste, goda masala, dry mango powder, coriander and jeera powder, salt and oats mix well. Due to wetness of spinach and potato the oats should be mixed well if required add some water. Make small tikkis of the mixture.
- Add some oil on non-stick pan and shallow fry the oats from both sides till it becomes crispy.
- Serve with pudina, coriander chutney or tamarind chutney.

## SOYABEAN KHEEMA

### Ingredients

- Soya granules – ½ katori
- Green peas – 2 tbsp.
- Onion – 2 no.
- Tomato – 1 no.
- Ginger garlic paste – 1 tbsp.
- Garam masala – ½ tbsp.
- Turmeric – 1 pinch
- Red chilies powder. – ½ tbsp.
- Bay leaf – 2 no.
- Milk – ¾ cup
- Cashew nuts – 10 gm
- Oil – 2 tbsp.
- Coriander leaves.

### Method

- Cook soya granules in mixture of milk and water for 20 mins.
- Chop onions and tomato, heat oil add bay leaf, ginger garlic paste, garam masala and chopped onions.
- Fry onions till it turns golden brown then add turmeric, red chilies and chopped tomato.
- Fry till oil oozes out then add cashew nut paste and soya granules. Add water place a lid and cook for 15-20 minutes. When it is cooked add boiled green peas and decorate with coriander leaves and serve hot.

## TOFU PALAK PUDINA PARATHA

### Ingredients

- Mix flour [wheat flour + soya flour]–2 cups
- Grated tofu – 1 cup
- Palak (Spinach) – 1 cup [finely chopped]
- Pudina leaves – ½ cup
- Red chilies powder. – 1 tbsp.
- Green chilies – 1 tbsp.
- Grated ginger – 1 tbsp.
- Chat masala – 1tbsp.
- Oil – 2 tbsp.
- Salt to taste

### Method

- Add heated oil in mix flour and prepare dough. Keep aside for 1 hour.
- For stuffing mix together grated tofu, finely chopped palak and pudina leaves, salt, red chilies powder and chat masala.
- Heat oil, add chopped green chilies, grated ginger and above mixture and fry the mixture for 5 minutes till it becomes dry.

- Make 2 chapatis of the prepared dough, spread the above mixture evenly on one chapatti place the other chapatti on it press a little and close it.
- Add 1 tbsp oil on nonstick pan roast the paratha from both sides and serve hot with curd.

# SUGGESTED READING

**Additional suggested reading for enthusiasts**

1. Annual Reviews of Diabetes.
2. Chronic Complications of Diabetes.
3. Clinical Diabetes: Translating Research into Practice.
4. Clinical Dietetics and Nutrition.
5. Diabetes from Research to Diagnosis and Treatment.
6. Difficult Diabetes.
7. Evidence-based Diabetes Care.
8. Ferri's Clinical Advisor-2009.
9. Handbook of Diabetes Foot.
10. International Textbook of Diabetes Mellitus - Vol. I and Vol. II.
11. Joslin's Textbook of Diabetes.
12. Novo Interactive Nutrition Assistant-NINA.
13. RSSDI Textbook of Diabetes Mellitus.
14. Staged Diabetes Management.
15. Textbook of Diabetes-Volume 1 and Volume 2.
16. Therapy for Diabetes and Related Disorders.

**The whole new world of Internet**

I sincerely thank all those who have written volumes on the various aspects of diabetes, for giving me an inspiration and guidelines while writing this concise book.

# INDEX

## D

## E



## F



## G

## H



## I

## U



## V



## W



## X



## Y